Body Sculpting with Kettlebells for Women

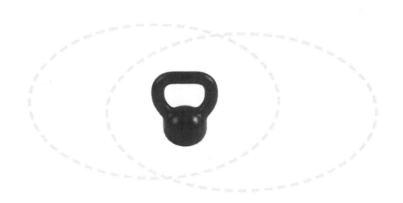

Lorna Kleidman

America's First International Master of Kettlebell Sport
Two-Time World Kettlebell Sport Champion

hatherleigh

BODY SCULPTING WITH KETTLEBELLS FOR WOMEN

Text copyright ©2009 Lorna Kleidman

Hatherleigh Press is committed to preserving and protecting the natural resources of the Earth. Environmentally responsible and sustainable practices are embraced within the company's mission statement.

Hatherleigh Press is a member of the Publishers Earth Alliance, committed to preserving and protecting the natural resources of the planet while developing a sustainable business model for the book publishing industry.

www.hatherleighpress.com

This book was edited, designed, and photographed in the village of Hobart, New York. Hobart is a community that has embraced books and publishing as a component of its livelihood. There are several unique bookstores in the village. For more information, please visit www.hobartbookvillage.com.

Library of Congress Cataloging-in-Publication Data

Kleidman, Lorna.
  Body sculpting with kettlebells for women: the complete exercise plan / Lorna Kleidman.
     p. cm.
  ISBN 978-1-57826-307-3 (pbk.: alk. paper) 1. Weight training. 2. Kettlebells. 3. Physical fitness for women. I. Title.
  GV546.K55 2009
  613.7'045--dc22

                    2009022189

Body Sculpting with Kettlebells for Women is available for bulk purchase, special promotions, and premiums. For information on reselling and special purchase opportunities, call 1-800-528-2550 and ask for the Special Sales Manager.

Cover Design by Nick Macagnone
Interior Design by Nick Macagnone
Photography by Catarina Astrom

10 9 8 7 6 5 4 3 2 1

DISCLAIMER

Consult your physician before beginning any exercise program. The author and publisher of this book and workout disclaim any liability, personal or professional, resulting from the misapplication of any of the training procedures described in this publication.

Dedication

For my Mom, Phyllis.

Many thanks to Daniela Denaro
for her participation as a model.

My unending gratitude to those who have
always brought out the best and continue
to inspire me—Adam Cronin, Michelle Khai,
Larry Twohig and, of course, Carl.

Body Sculpting *with* **Kettlebells**

Table of Contents

Introduction

As a child growing up in New York, I was far from athletic. Bouts of exercise-induced asthma were practically routine, as much a part of my daily experience as getting out of bed. My lung capacity was so weak that I was unable to keep up with friends and classmates when playing basketball, volleyball or simply running around during tag at recess. After a few minutes into any game, I would be predictably hunched over, struggling to catch my breath as I watched my teammates continue to play without me. Unfortunately, that was simply the norm for me when it came to recreational activities. I just did what I could.

Yet, although my participation time was often limited, I actually enjoyed scholastic sports. I would not be dissuaded from playing with my friends or being active. The way I saw it, I simply had no choice. Still, it would take decades before I developed any kind of physical stamina.

At age fourteen, I began to study dance. Soon, I was thriving. The format of the classes enabled me to catch my breath while the teacher demonstrated new steps. My love affair with dance lasted for years and helped me navigate the awkward teen years. Although it was thrilling to perform in professional musicals, I knew theater would not be the right long-term career choice for me.

In 1991 I obtained a license in massage therapy. I immediately began to build a thriving private practice while continuing my education by studying many forms of bodywork including ART (Active Release Technique), an innovative form of soft tissue therapy used by athletes and non-athletes alike.

With my dance shoes now in the back of the closet, I joined a local gym, yearning to get back into some form of regular physical activity. At that point, most of my time was spent with free weights and machines, yet I was frequently fascinated by the sight of the drenched, gloriously exhausted aerobics-class participants exiting the fitness studio each day. Finally, thoroughly bored with the monotony of the weight machines, I gave the class a try.

It turned out that high-impact aerobics, with its fast and continuous pace, was a revelation for me. The classes were at once inspiring and humbling, since each day I would have to stop every 3 or 4 minutes to use my asthma inhaler and catch my breath.

I relegated myself to the back of the studio for much of the first year because I could not keep up with women twice my age. Yet the class's energy, pulsating music and motivation of the instructor fueled my desire to try to keep up with the other participants and motivated me to return to the class 3 days per week.

A full year passed before I was finally able to make it through the hour of aerobics class without stopping. Little did I know that this was to be my first step on the road to overcoming life-long debilitating asthma and becoming a competitive athlete. Encouraged by this first real glimmer of my physical potential, I challenged myself further by enrolling in step classes, kickboxing and traditional boxing training. I had always enjoyed exercise, but now that my lungs were able to keep up with the rest of my body, there was no stopping me. Gradually, over a five-year period, I was able to perform as well as my gym peers for the first time in my life.

Until the day in 2005 when I first picked up a kettlebell, I thought I had formulated the perfect exercise regimen of weight training, cardio and conditioning. I had a very specific weekly routine that I was devoted to. However, the reality that I soon discovered was that my fitness regimen was in control of me.

I had become the typical fitness-class junkie, working out two hours each weekday and four hours every Saturday. I was painfully afraid of gaining weight or losing the conditioning I had worked so hard for. I resented any obligation or social plans that might take me away from my routine. Thinking that my way was the only way to stay fit, I never could have imagined that there was an effective way to work out that didn't require hours and days in the gym. Everything about my life was to change the day I picked up a kettlebell.

In 2005, I moved to South Florida, where I treated myself to a personal training session at a local gym. Interestingly, the person I chose just happened to specialize in kettlebell training. By this time, I had participated in some very demanding workout classes and was very familiar with using weights, but the challenge posed by the kettlebell took me completely by surprise.

The first thing I noticed was the speed at which my heart rate increased within the first few minutes of learning the kettlebell swing, getting my cardio fired up early in the workout.

Immediately hooked on this new fitness tool, I quickly shifted the focus of my workouts to learning and practicing the skills of kettlebell movements. Within a couple of weeks, I experienced something I had never felt before: as I moved, I could actually feel the deepest layer muscles of my spine and abdominal region. These are muscles I had only known of through schematics in massage therapy manuals, but now they were becoming awakened, as I experienced the differences between muscles of movement and muscles of stabilization. These kettlebell workouts were recruiting the deepest levels of muscle, tendons and ligaments and it felt incredible!

These were results I could not only feel, but could also see! My physique was becoming leaner and more defined than ever before, heavier weights were easier to lift and my jumping ability had become more explosive and easier, without jumping (plyometrics) as an integral part of my kettlebell training. Most importantly, my lung capacity was becoming less of an issue and my overall endurance was increasing. Finally, the act of breathing, a primary hindrance since childhood, was coming naturally to me and I didn't have to scramble to use my inhaler every few minutes. I experienced the glory of being 'winded' as opposed to struggling to breathe at all.

By the time I reached my mid-30's, I began to notice an increase in my metabolism— when most women in that age bracket face new difficulty maintaining their once slender waistline and thighs. My high metabolism was thanks to kettlebells, and my new workout routine—a mere 1 hour per day, 4-5 days a week schedule—was liberation compared to the rigid 6 days a week, 2 hours a day routine I had before. I began to see my ideal body being realized. Working out with kettlebells dramatically increased my metabolism within the first month, to the extent that I could again enjoy bread, pasta or even dessert a few times each week. After a love-hate battle with these foods for years, I could finally eat them again. This continues to this day; now, when carbs and sweets are on my plate, I don't have to feel guilty about it!

In 2007 I traveled to San Diego to learn authentic competitive Russian kettlebell lifting as part of a certified course. At the end of the curriculum, participants are required to demonstrate proficiency by completing a pre-determined number of lifts. Unbeknownst to me, I surpassed the required reps necessary for the first qualifier toward international competition! As it turns out, the competition was to be held in eight months, so I decided to join the team to represent the USA in the 15th International Girevoy Sport Championships. At the event I proudly became the first American to earn the title Master of Sport International Level (MSIL). I was also thrilled to win both Gold and Silver medals in my age and weight category respectively. The following year, at the 2008 International Championship, in Chatillon, Italy, I earned two Gold medals.

But my greatest satisfaction comes from teaching others about the amazing qualities of the kettlebell. Currently, in addition to competing, I teach semi-private classes in New York City with students of all fitness levels and ages, including children, teens and adults.

One of my students had just given birth to her second child when we met. She expressed her desire to start 'something new,' as she was tired of her previous exercise routine. After 2 months in my class she called with excitement:

"My back used to ache every day from lifting the kids, leaning over to change them, getting them in and out of the car seat, making the beds…all the simple day–to-day stuff would wear me out. But now I'm beginning to feel so much more strength and ability in myself, as if my body's not letting me down any longer. Now I know how to use my body to move objects in the proper way, so it's easy and doesn't cause strain. Lifting or carrying the kids isn't so difficult any more—and I'm getting as lean as I was before I got married!"

Some of my adult students are in their 70's! The kettlebell is perfect for all age ranges and fitness levels.

My story of physical change can be yours, too! I am stronger, leaner, have more endurance and look better than I did 10 years ago—even though I now do less exercising. In addition, qualities so important for atheletes, including balance, shifting weight quickly, and hand-eye coordination, have also been enhanced, without the need for performing sport-specific drills. Today the asthma that plagued me is practically non-existent.

Whether you want to eliminate cellulite,

achieve strong, healthy bones and joints, improve body awareness and balance, or improve your posture and flexibility, all of these benefits can be achieved with less time spent exercising. You too can eat healthfully, but eat what you want and never stress over missing a workout. What liberation this is! You can enjoy weeklong vacations without having to negotiate or even consider gym time. What more could you ask for from a fitness tool?

Now it's time for you to begin your own journey...

Introducing Kettlebells Part I

What Sets the Kettlebell Apart?

1

The History of Kettlebells: From Ancient Marketplace to Modern Day Phenomenon

The kettlebell has an unusual history. In many Eastern European countries in the 1800's, kettlebells in varying sizes were used as counter-weights on scales in the marketplace. For fun, vendors and farmers would show off their strength and prowess by pressing, swinging or tossing the weights about.

As generations passed, these casual movements developed into technical lifts requiring skill, which fathers taught to their sons.

Called 'giris' in Russian, kettlebells soon evolved into a popular pastime in Russian culture, with lifting and juggling exhibitions becoming standard features at fairs, during holiday times, and as part of circus acts.

It wasn't long before the Soviet Union recognized the multiple benefits kettlebells would provide the numerous men and women who worked as laborers in the USSR economy.

Originally perceived as an entertaining pastime, kettlebells were soon recognized as an incomparable exercise tool since they were readily available, mobile, and indestructible.

The ongoing popularity of kettlebells led to the formation in 1981 of the first Kettlebell Commission. The Commission enforced mandatory kettlebell exercise and conditioning for the populous, with the understanding that this singular instrument would keep the country's people fit, increase productivity, and decrease healthcare costs. Kettlebells subsequently became the conditioning tool of choice for the Russian Special Forces, creating

Kettlebells were soon recognized as an incomparable exercise tool since they were readily available, mobile, and indestructible.

soldiers who possessed incredible strength and endurance, and for the Soviet Olympic weightlifting team who for decades have dominated the sport.

Kettlebells first arrived in the United States in the 1920's with Russian immigrants, but were never exposed to the broader U.S. populace. Instead, the primary users were Russian devotees and some weightlifters. When the American fitness craze first took hold in the 1970's, there emerged a proliferation of mega-gyms, promising quick-fix workouts. Fancy equipment, which included shiny thousand-dollar machines and single muscle group gadgets, eclipsed the need for skilled professional trainers. Like most big businesses, as fitness in America became a booming industry, its objective was not based on the overall health and longevity of the individual, but rather on the monetary science of membership statistics and marketing. Kettlebells were considered antiquated, simplistic, and far too "low-tech" for the modern age. Nothing

Kettlebell workouts bring about **real results, real fast!**

could have been further from the truth.

With the coming and going of the various fitness trends that focused on simple, glitzy workouts, the last several years have brought about a tremendous appreciation of functional training, including the use of familiar training tools such as Swiss and medicine balls. As a result, kettlebells have emerged and are now recognized worldwide as the superior tool for multi-planar functional training, making two-

dimensional movement patterns such as those performed with body bars seem useless.

Kettlebell workouts bring about real results, real fast!

How Kettlebells Got Their Name

Surprisingly, we turn to the church for the genesis of the kettlebell's name, but first we must go even farther back and visit the history of the dumbbell.

For centuries, church bells were rung through the laborious act of pulling levers, which were strung through wheels and attached to the bells. The largest bells weighed as much as three tons, requiring a team of qualified men possessing great strength, skill and coordination to achieve the proper sound. In an effort to perfect their technique, bell-ringers would practice with silent, non-clapper bells called 'dumb-bells'. Athletes then took advantage of the concept that bells came in different weights and sizes, ingeniously attaching two small bells to the ends of a wooden or metal bar (barbell) or utilizing the detached clapper as a tool to increase muscle size and strength. As athletes began to create purpose-built equipment, the name 'dumbbell' remained.

Similarly, Scottish legend has it that would-be strongmen and athletes utilized old or leaky cast iron cooking kettles as rudimentary weights. Back in the day, nothing was wasted! By filling the kettles with sand, soil, or lead shot, they became load-adjustable strength-training tools which could be lifted, pulled or swung about. In time, the name 'kettle-bell' was coined.

Although now we know the modern versions of dumbbells and kettlebells, in fact weights with handles have been around for millennia, going back to ancient Greek and Roman times.

Dumbbells vs. Kettlebells

To sum it up, the difference between a dumbbell and a kettlebell is the difference between a conventional workout and one that is optimally effective, efficient, and long-lasting. Again, it's the results that make the difference.

Sculpting the body with dumbbells involves an exhaustive list of separate body part exercises, with the emphasis on larger muscle groups or highly visible "vanity" areas. This often means neglecting many other not so visible, but equally important, areas that are vital to postural integrity and functional movement.

> A dynamic kettlebell vs. a static dumbbell is the difference between:
>
> A rip-roaring roller coaster and a child's playground swing
>
> A satisfying gourmet meal and a bland TV dinner
>
> High-Def plasma screen entertainment and an old-fashioned picture tube television set.

Let's imagine the following example:

In an effort to become well-toned, more graceful, and more coordinated, you've signed up for a series of dance lessons. Each lesson begins with arm movements, followed by some instructions on how to perform various steps finally ending with a few stretches.

Although you will probably learn the fundamentals of dance, the steps—the movements—are never so united that you are actually dancing. Conventional resistance training is approached in a similar manner.

In the last century the fitness industry has largely taught us to divide the body into an inventory of muscles to be trained, as opposed

Exercise will become **enjoyable again**, just as when you played as a child.

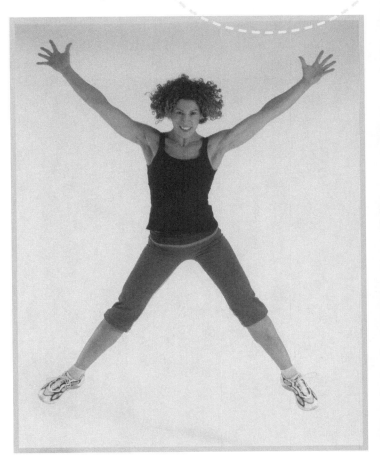

to movements to be mastered. The dual benefit of movement within stabilization is the hallmark of kettlebell sculpting, making it the most efficient and effective tool for meeting your fitness goals.

Kettlebells provide complete physical fitness through three-dimensional, whole body movements. You will sculpt every muscle, working from the deep (skeletal) to the superficial (what you see in the mirror), all while you enjoy the challenging, free-flowing movements this unique tool allows. Exercise will become enjoyable again, just as when you played as a child.

As your muscles become toned, these same exercises will enable you to be more efficient in your daily activities, protect you from injury, and in many cases even hasten rehabilitation.

So ask yourself, why workout to create a sports car body when you still have a cheap under-powered engine inside?

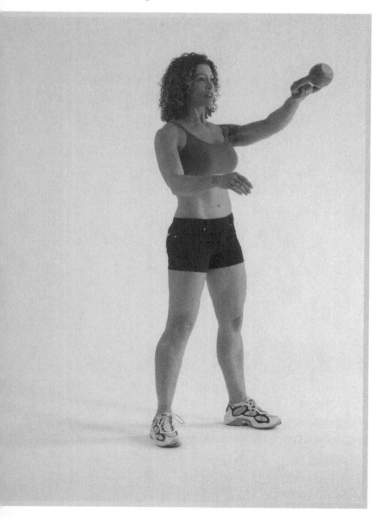

How the Unique Design of the Kettlebell Handle Distinguishes it from Dumbbells, Body Bars and Medicine Balls

Unlike most resistance tools, the kettlebell's weight is displaced beyond the center of the hand, challenging the user to control its movements while simultaneously counter-balancing its resistance through large ranges of motion. The handle creates an additional joint on your arm, producing a variable center of gravity depending upon how you swing, push or pull it.

In addition, kettlebells allow for natural rotational movements which are performed in exercises such as the Figure 8 (see page 77) and Russian Twist (see page 98), which are not possible with dumbbells.

Dumbbell features:	Kettlebell features:
Centered in the palm, allowing only two-dimensional movement	Handle creates variable three-dimensional movement
Unnaturally even distribution of weight	Round shape
Horizontal plane	Vertical center of gravity (enhances natural movement patterns)

The Amazing Kettlebell Swing

The swing is a fundamental kettlebell movement that is initiated by flexion and extension of the hips. As the bell rises on the upswing, your body will naturally engage your entire core, defined as everything from your chest to your knees, in order to counter-act the momentary forward pull of the kettlebell. Once the bell reaches chest height, it will suddenly feel weightless before gravity initiates its downswing. Here, your body will naturally stabilize itself while following the bell as it passes through your legs and you power the upswing once again.

Without ever having to "crunch your abs" or work until you "feel the burn", your body will simultaneously and organically engage the core musculature and the prime movers at all times in order to maintain your center of gravity. You'll experience these engagements occurring without conscious effort, as you counter-act the bell's velocity.

Compare the Kettlebell Swing vs. a Dumbbell to Achieve the Same Results:

Let's say your primary fitness goal is to tone and sculpt your legs, butt, and abs, for an upcoming beach vacation.

The kettlebell swing provides an unparalleled range of motion as its momentum is powered upward and followed downward.

Muscles sculpted in one exercise with a kettlebell

- **Glutes**: All sections of the gluteus, including maximus, medius and minimus (the muscles that when sculpted, give the nice indentation on the side of the butt)
- **Hamstrings:** Work with the glutes to bring the hips into full extension for a powerful, authoritative stride
- **Inner thighs:** Aid in powering upswing

and support on downswing

- **Quadriceps:** Aid in powering upswing and support on downswing
- **Calves:** Aid in powering upswing and support on downswing
- **Abs:** Both deep and superficial layers of abdominal muscles engage on the upswing as well as the downswing to stabilize the spine and counteract the bell's movements. Obliques are greatly utilized during Single Arm Swings and overhead positions.
- **Back:** The erector spinae, quadratus lumborum and the very deep multifidus are constantly engaged, bringing the body upright when the bell is at its highest and also act as stabilizing muscles on the downswing.
- **Middle and lower trapezius, rhomboids, latissimus dorsi:** Muscles that retract the shoulder and arm are employed at the top of the swing, toning and strengthening the upper back. Synchronization of muscles occurs to create fluid movement.
- **Grip:** The grip is always strengthened when using a kettlebell. A strong grip is useful in all sports as well as daily activities. How difficult is it to open a jar of spaghetti sauce!?

All the muscle groups listed are constantly engaged, contracting, relaxing, shortening, lengthening, responding and working together in synchronicity, making kettlebell body-sculpting an intense and effective way to reach your goals. It is the intensity that creates the fast changes, so that you recognize results in less time.

Remember, the swing is but one example of how you can sculpt multiple muscle groups in just one exercise, requiring just 5 to 10 minutes of your session!

Body Sculpting *with* **Kettlebells**

Now let's take a look at what's required to achieve the same results with a dumbbell:

Dumbbell

- 🔔 Squats for gluteals and quadriceps
- 🔔 Dead Lifts for hamstrings
- 🔔 Lateral Lunges for inner thighs and gluteus medius/minimus
- 🔔 Calf Raises
- 🔔 Leg Raises and Crunches for abdominals
- 🔔 Extensions for erector spinae and quadratus lumborum

I don't know about you, but this would take me an hour to get through, **BUT WE ARE NOT DONE YET!**

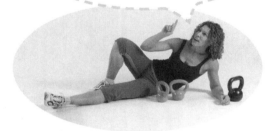

- 🔔 Bent Over Row for trapezius and rhomboid
- 🔔 Wrist Curls for grip
- 🔔 A few Jump Squats for ballistic power, which is present in the majority of kettlebell movements.

But wait! The cardiovascular component is missing.

No amount of dumbbell lifting will get your heart rate stimulated like the kettlebell, so get on the treadmill or bicycle for a few sprints to make up the "cardio" portion of your workout.

Doesn't this seem like a lot of work and a lot of time spent when you could be doing something fun? The dumbbell approach is akin to a program for a one-hour training session whereas you'll see in this book's series of programs, the swing takes only 5 to 10 minutes of your 45 minute session, giving you ultimate results in less time!

Benefits of a
Kettlebell Workout

2

The Kettlebell's Shape Enables an Endless Variety of Movement Patterns

As anyone who has embarked on a physical fitness quest well knows, variety is the key to sticking with a regimen.

The kettlebell will give you infinite freedom of movement. As you begin to swing it, you will notice that the kettlebell seems to come alive! And your instincts are right—it is alive with momentum, traveling in the direction you intend it to go, continuing until you slow or stop it.

The constant start, stop and simultaneous multidimensional resistance sets the kettlebell apart from all other resistance tools.

The kettlebell's handle features a distinctive design that allows fluid hand-to-hand passing, enabling an unlimited variety of dynamic exercises. The handle also permits you to create large ranges of motion, rotational patterns, swings and the unique ability to transition in and out of various exercises quickly and safely. In time, you will likely create your own signature moves to challenge yourself!

Kettlebell movements mimic real-life movement patterns that are natural to the human body, reducing the risk of injury.

Application to Daily Living

If you were to consider your daily activities and their required movements (walking, reaching, carrying for example), you would agree that most of your routine activities require some form of lifting, pulling, pushing or balancing objects that are not centered in the palm of your hand (with the exception of a cell phone!).

Here are a few examples of activities involving displaced center of gravity:

- Walking a dog
- Carrying grocery bags
- Moving furniture
- Swinging a golf club or tennis racquet
- Partner dancing
- Surfing

Logistical Benefits of the Kettlebell Sculpt

CONVENIENCE AND DURABILITY: Kettlebells are indestructible and require very little space.

They can be brought to the office, kept in the home, garage, basement or even left outside. Inclement weather or temperature changes will not cause damage.

AFFORDABILITY: The purchase of three starter kettlebells is an investment in a virtual full-spectrum home gym, the price of which is equivalent to two month's membership at most gyms.

VERSATILITY: Kettlebells allow for a mix of grinds and ballistic movements so that you acquire both static and dynamic strength. Grinds are slow movements that teach the body to adapt to overall tension, whereas ballistic movements require short bursts of muscular activity at faster rates of speed which utilize the elastic characteristics of muscles, tendons and ligaments. Running, throwing, and jumping are examples of ballistic actions. A ball thrown with a full wind-up results in a longer throw than if you were to throw without a wind-up. Kettlebell sculpting offers all the benefits of ballistic movements—power, speed, agility and reduction in body fat—but without impact to the joints.

TIME EFFICIENCY: Workout sessions can be effective in as little as 15 minutes, making the kettlebell the "no excuses" tool of choice!

PERFORMANCE STUDY: Sergey Voropayev, Ph.D (in 1983) observed the physical training of two groups of college students over a period of a few years. A standard battery of the armed forces physical training tests was used: pull-ups, a standing broad jump, a 100m sprint, and a 1K run. The control group followed the typical university physical training program which was military oriented and emphasized the above exercises. The experimental group just lifted kettlebells. In spite of the lack of practice on the tested drills, the kettlebell group achieved better scores in every single category than their standard-trained counterparts.

- Catching yourself so as not to slip or trip
- Handling an open umbrella during a storm

Another common example is lifting a child. A child's shifting weight is not easy to manage, even when they are asleep. And when they are moving about, you must manage a weight that is both active and displaced. This is what kettlebells are all about—as its momentum pulls it away, you counter by pulling it toward you. As the weight is pushed or swung overhead, you immediately establish your center of gravity and stabilize.

High Pull with Kettlebell

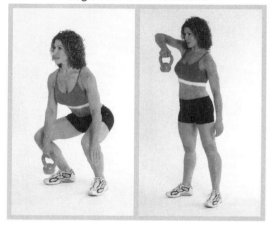

High Pull movement utilized to lift heavy luggage

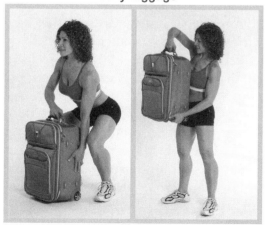

Injury Prevention

In life and in sports, most injuries occur during the deceleration phase of a movement, as in landing from a jump, walking down a flight of stairs, or suddenly stopping short. Because of the dynamic nature of their movement patterns, kettlebells condition the body for deceleration as well as acceleration. In order to slow or stop the momentum of the bell, opposing muscle groups must quickly respond, fostering and reestablishing healthy, stable joints.

Kettlebell sculpting will create and reinforce strong muscles and bones, conditioning them statically and dynamically from every angle, while maintaining your center of gravity.

For example, the offset center of gravity ultimately enhances shoulder joint flexibility, stability and strength. Your core, defined as everything from your chest to your knees, will become the supportive functional structure it is meant to be, eliminating muscle aches due to poor posture. Your upper back, including your neck, will become strong and stable, eliminating chronic discomfort due to weakened musculature.

To achieve the same benefits that kettlebell sculpting yields, you would have to engage in power lifting for strength and speed, yoga for dynamic flexibility and kickboxing for intense cardio. One regimen versus three. Which would you prefer?

Results Attained Through Kettlebell Sculpting

Today, it is rare to encounter someone who is not trying to squeeze more into the same 24-hour day that once seemed like plenty of time. Everyone now is in a time crunch, which brings me to the number one benefit of kettlebell sculpting: Your hard work is rewarded rapidly!

Kettlebells will change your body FAST! You will literally feel yourself transition from fat storing to fat burning in just a few sessions. The results of kettlebell sculpting are supported by studies showing that short bursts of intense

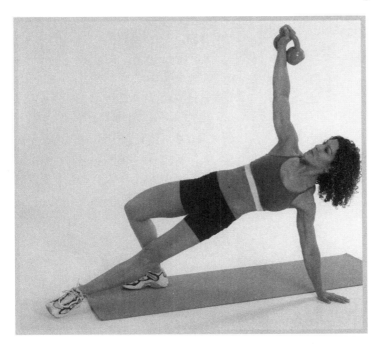

exercises will stoke your metabolism for up to 24 hours after the workout; in fact, with the kettlebell, your metabolism will burn for days after consistent workouts, allowing you to enjoy days off from workouts while your metabolism is still burning away!

Here's what you can look forward to:

Cosmetic Results

- A firm, round and lifted butt
- Reduced, slimmer waistline
- Flatter stomach and abdomen
- Leaner thighs
- Fat loss
- Toned and more defined muscles
- Muscular symmetry
- Improved posture, especially for the often underused and neglected upper back
- Reduction of cellulite
- Tighter stomach and core following pregnancy

Performance/Physiological Results

- Increased energy
- Increased aerobic/anaerobic capacity and reduction in both active and resting heart rate
- Optimized lung function
- Improved hand-eye coordination, timing and spatial awareness
- Enhanced Pilates and/or yoga performance
- Enhanced reaction time and better speed
- Improved balance and coordination
- Enhanced grip strength
- More effective rehabilitation
- Enhanced joint stability
- Enhanced or maintained bone density
- Elimination of muscular imbalances

Psychological Results

The programs in *Body Sculpting with Kettlebells* are progressively challenging and mentally engaging, requiring you to be in the moment. The primary mental benefit is better concentration and a higher level of awareness.

- Kettlebells are fun, dynamic and stimulating
- You will look forward to working out instead of dreading it
- You can reduce time spent working out
- You will be more easily satisfied as your desired results will be seen and felt quickly
- You will move with confidence, energy, and authority

About the **Workouts**

Part II

Before your Workout

3

Safety

To achieve the best results from your kettlebell workouts, follow this book's step-by-step instructions, and adhere to these guidelines:

1. **Consult with your doctor** before beginning this or any new fitness regimen.

2. **Wrist bands:** The kettlebell is a constantly shifting variable weight. Many drills begin or end with the bell 'settling' on the back of your wrist. A pair of wrist sweatbands are perfect to cushion your wrists. With practice, you will develop the timing necessary for precise, intentional and smooth landings.

3. **Footwear:** Cross-trainers or tennis shoes that have flat, thin soles and provide lateral stability are favorable since they will provide the stability necessary to maintain your body's center of gravity. Practicing in bare feet is not recommended.

4. **Gloves:** Ladies, you CAN go without! Gloves will diminish the sensation in the hand, which is vital for proper feedback and responsiveness in managing the bell's ever shifting movements.

   Your hands are the critical link in kettlebell lifting. They will become very strong, and who doesn't need strong hands?

   For some, calluses will naturally form with kettlebell use, particularly below the fingers at the top of the palm. This is a good thing, and the first sign that you are becoming a true kettlebell athlete. Calluses are easy to manage and no one will notice them, unless, like many kettlebell enthusiasts, you take pride and want to show them off! I'll leave that up to you!

5. **Hand Maintenance:** After a shower or bath, use a coarse nail file to buff your calluses flat and smooth. This should be done every two or three days.

   Keep nails on the shorter side to avoid brushing them against the kettlebell's handle as it rotates.

6. **Always eat something light** 60-90 minutes prior to your workout. Unlike yoga or cardio which can be performed on an empty stomach, kettlebell sculpting requires much more energy from your system as a whole, so be sure to add some fuel before you begin.

7. **Always prepare your body and mind** with the recommended warm-up and recover with a proper cool down.

8. **Do not take your skills for granted!** Approach each session with a clear mind, dedicated to the day's program, taking your kettlebell regimen seriously. Talking, multi-tasking, or watching TV during your workout jeopardizes your safety. Your time with the kettlebell is the one thing in your day you will do in a manner that is entirely focused and dedicated to the moment. If you cannot focus on the skills of the movements while performing them, find another time or another day to do your session because the rare instances when injuries or accidents occur are the result of the lifter not paying attention.

9. **Learn to "bring down" safely:** If there comes a moment when you feel you cannot maintain the kettlebell in an overhead position, use both hands to guide it to the rack position or down to the ground, maintaining flexion from your hips and keeping your back flat.

   If you cannot maintain a swinging movement and want to bring it down, slow the momentum using both hands, always maintaining hip flexion and a flat back.

10. **Personal space:** Be aware of your 'behind'! If using the kettlebell in a tight space (which is not recommended but is sometimes unavoidable), be aware of the total circumference. Make sure there are no people, children or pets that may potentially walk up from behind or cross

in front of you. Do not swing the kettlebell in front of a TV, furniture or other destructible objects. If you are in a public place, use objects to define your space.

11. **Workout on dry, flat, surfaces.** If you are on grass, check the ground for uneven areas before moving about. For advanced workouts, sand is wonderfully challenging if you have the opportunity to try it!

12. **No hand lotion prior to training.**

13. **Listen to your body.** If you have a tendency to be overly enthusiastic or to over-train, this point is for you! Even though you want to keep doing more to push yourself... DON'T! Use the days in between the workouts to recover. Getting adequate rest and nutrition will help your body adapt and change, as well as serve your next workout session. If you get the itch to do some form of activity on the off days, choose a short run, jump rope, yoga or Pilates. You will reap greater rewards by pacing yourself according to the program, ensuring continued good performance on subsequent workouts without symptoms of over-training such as fatigue, loss of energy, insomnia, depression, chronic muscle or joint pain, or dehydration.

Your Workout Needs

Which Weights to Begin With

Keep in mind that kettlebell sculpting is quite unique. Do not make the mistake of thinking about it in the same frame of reference as other exercise regimens.

The suggested weight for each exercise should not be confused with other resistance tools such as dumbbells or medicine balls. A 15 lb kettlebell is not the same as a 15 lb dumbbell and you will notice the difference as soon as you begin moving it; this is when the 'real feel' becomes apparent. Just as we consider the weather in terms of actual temperature versus the 'real feel', kettlebells' actual weight differs from their 'real feel'. The 'real feel' of a 15 lb kettlebell in motion is only 5 or 6 lbs! The difference in weight perception is due to the presence of momentum.

Each program day offers the weight suggestion(s) for that workout. Each woman is different in ability and in strength, so you'll need to experiment a bit in the beginning.

As you become familiar with the various drills and their combinations, choose a weight with which you can perform 10 reps.

If 10 reps prove to be easy, use a weight that is 5 lbs heavier. As you progress with the program, you will begin to feel confident with particular movements. This is also a good time to challenge yourself with a heavier bell, increasing the weight by 5 lbs, depending on the weights available to you. Keep in mind that a heavier weight requires more exacting technique; review and follow the points laid out for each exercise to ensure proper movement and safety. When you are easily able to swing a bell for 25 reps, or press it for 10 reps in 3 separate sets, you will be ready to go up 5 lbs in weight. You may also choose to ease into a heavier weight by using it for only one of the listed sets of any exercise.

Who Should Get a Doctor's Permission?

It is vital that you visit a medical professional prior to beginning this program if you fit any of these categories:

- Significantly overweight
- Have high blood pressure
- Suffer from any heart condition
- Have any problems with balance (either due to skeletal, musculature, or inner-ear problems)
- Joint injury in the past 12 months
- Are currently pregnant
- Are over the age of 55

Note: Arthritis is not a contra-indication to kettlebell workouts, but be sure to warm-up thoroughly and listen to your body.

Here's all you'll need to get started:

The Basics	One 15 lb and one 20 lb kettlebell
A Smart Set	One of each 15, 20, 25 lb
Your comparative buying guide:	9 lb = 4 kg
	13 lb = 6 kg
	18 lb = 8 kg
	26 lb = 12 kg
	35 lb = 16 kg
	44 lb = 20 kg
	53 lb = 24 kg

Begin by acknowledging your limitations so you can safely exceed them!

Getting the Most
Out of Your Workout

4

Making the Program Work for You

The *Body Sculpting with Kettlebells* Program is effective and efficient, presenting progressive workouts that build in complexity and intensity so you avoid the plateaus often encountered in other fitness modalities. By following the book's program you will learn precise kettlebell skills in a safe and comprehensive manner while enhancing your strength, endurance, balance, coordination and so much more!

The following are variables that may be adjusted depending on your workout needs.

Frequency

After any form of exercise, your body undergoes a process of repairing and restoring. The frequency of the *Body Sculpting with Kettlebells* Program is designed to provide a balance between the stress placed on your body and the designated time allowed for recovery. Recovery days are as valuable as workout days as this is when your body goes through the physiological changes necessary to create a beautifully sculpted body.

You may perform the program 5 days per week provided you are familiar with the movements, are not sore from previous workouts and have proper nutrition.

You may perform the program a minimum 3 days per week if you are new to exercise or have not exercised in over a year.

Intensity

The human body is not meant to endure long periods of physical stress, particularly when it comes to resistance training. The more intense the workout, the shorter the duration should be –60 minutes maximum with rest periods of 90 seconds to 2 minutes maximum. Research shows that individuals in their 60's and 70's maintain strength, agility and overall health by increasing the intensity and decreasing the duration of their workouts.

Rep

A rep or repetition is the number of times you perform a movement. For example, if the assignment is 10 Squat/Press, you will squat with the kettlebell, then press it overhead to complete one rep. For movements like the Russian Twist (see page 98), moving the bell from your right side to your left and back again constitutes one rep.

Sets

A set represents how many times you complete a given number of repetitions of a particular exercise or group of exercises.

Rest Period

Rest period is the amount of time you have to recover after completing the reps in a set. Pay close attention to your resting time and do not allow yourself to get distracted. The rest periods that accompany each day's session will fluctuate from session to session. The 'light' days, which allow 30 – 45 seconds rest, should be just enough to glance at the next exercise and take a sip of

you have taken the first and most important step toward changing your body and your life.

water, then get back to sculpting!

Longer rest periods are given on heavier days to provide the necessary muscular recovery for the subsequent exercises.

Drills that indicate one side then the other, such as '8 each', mean the exercise should be performed on both sides before taking a rest.

Supersets are presented throughout the program. This is when you will perform two different drills consecutively, resting after they are completed.

If days one through four prove to be very challenging, stay with these first few workouts for an additional week before moving to week two so that you build the foundation for what's ahead. Stick with it and be patient. You should find the workouts to be challenging and leave you a bit sore. After all, you are utilizing many of your muscle groups at one time, through large ranges of motion—a totally new experience for your body! Rest assured, after a couple of weeks the initial soreness will be a faint memory.

The Gold Program (see page 139) will introduce timed sets utilizing a clock instead of counting reps. These timed sets will also be shorter but more intense sessions than those performed within the week.

The Platinum Program (see page 169) will seamlessly join many of the elementary movements so that the sets are longer.

Training for Fat Loss

Whether your goal is to trim down for health reasons, an upcoming event or to feel better about yourself, realize that you have taken the first and most important step toward changing your body and your life by following the *Body Sculpting with Kettlebells* Program!

As women, we continually face a variety of factors that challenge us in our quest to be fit. Genetics plays a major role in the makeup of who we are physically, as does time of life, levels of stress and nutrition to name but a few.

Remember that throughout any physical

process your overall health is your first priority. Don't get caught up in how big or small a particular body part looks or disrespect your body with binges or deprivation.

Your fitness journey should be a process that challenges you while at the same time is rewarding and fun. A process of daily choices as opposed to a final destination; make it a journey of self-discovery by asking yourself, "How far can I go with this today?" "Do I have what it takes to create the body that I know I have inside?"

Of course you do; now make it happen!

Once you begin the program and realize progress, you will have newfound respect for your body's innate capability, so that while you may admire another woman's physique, you are also proud and comfortable in your own body, which is now transforming as a result of your commitment to your goals.

Focus on the reasons you want to look your best, the image of yourself as you know you can be—lean, strong, confident and feeling good about yourself.

The best way for active individuals to lose fat is by increasing the intensity or duration of exercise while simultaneously cutting down on calories. The former is easily accomplished by adhering to the program, the latter is detailed in the nutrition section.

Now let's look at some practical ideas that will help you to reach your goals:

- Make exercise a non-negotiable part of your day. If you are in a time crunch, do one of Saturday's short and intense workouts—you'll always be glad you did!
- Post a picture of the body you would like to aspire to on your refrigerator door, in your bathroom and on a full length mirror. You may also keep wallet size prints of this picture in your car and purse to inspire and remind you to stay on course.
- Nurture friendships that are mutually supportive
- Workout with a friend
- Workout to music that you love
- Believe in yourself

The Reality

There's no need to follow any particular diet in order to reach and maintain your sculpted body.

Here's what you need to do to lose fat:

- Follow the *Body Sculpting with Kettlebells* program of workouts
- Eat healthfully as indicated in the nutrition section
- Become aware of your portions and do not overeat
- Eat your last meal no later than 3 hours prior to bedtime

If you can incorporate these four principles into your lifestyle, you'll be on your way to permanent fat loss, strength, confidence and a gorgeous body!

The Fundamentals of Fat Loss Include:

1. Increased Metabolism
   - Workout consistently
   - Lift weights
   - Burn more calories than you consume

2. Nutrition
   - Eat at the right times of the day
   - Eat five or six small meals per day

- Eat small amounts of good fats
- Eat natural foods, no processed or fried foods
- Eat plenty of complex carbs, fruits and vegetables
- Eat lean protein

The more demand on the muscles, the more calories are burned. **The more calories are burned, the more fat is lost.**

3. Visualize Yourself as You Would Like to Be
Remember that overeating is still overeating, even if you're consuming nothing but "natural and healthy" foods, but you knew that!

Burn Calories = Lose Fat

The more intense the workout session, the more demand will be placed on the muscles. When the muscles are working, the body burns more calories, regardless of the activity you are participating in. Keep in mind that cardiovascular activities, such as running, only burn calories while you are performing the activity, whereas a kettlebell workout offers the intensity of multi-muscle group involvement, resulting in the loss of unwanted fat. In addition, the lean muscle acquired will continue to burn calories long after your workout is over, so even at rest your metabolism is stoked!

The more demand on the muscles, the more calories are burned. The more calories are burned, the more fat is lost.

Training for Strength

Resistance training is the fastest way to improve muscle strength and endurance. Some misconceptions associated with resistance training are that women will develop bulging muscles; in fact, women do not naturally possess the hormones necessary to build the kind of muscle mass that men possess. Rest assured, if a man were to train with this book's program of workouts, he too would burn fat and build lean muscle. This result is due to the unique characteristics of the kettlebell and the program's design.

The truth is that muscle burns up to five times as many calories at rest compared to fat, so the more muscle you have, the more calories you will burn, and the more likely it is that you will maintain your new physique.

The *Body Sculpting with Kettlebells* program is specifically designed to build strength while burning fat. But strength means more than just strong muscles; this program also creates stronger connective tissues such as tendons and ligaments that increase joint stability, range of motion, and bone density and reduce the risk of injuries.

Divide and Conquer

Research has shown that performing three or four 15-minute workouts is just as effective as performing one 45 to 60-minute workout session. The *Body Sculpting with Kettlebells* program can be easily divided into separate workout sessions that suit your timetable, making it the perfect solution for your busy schedule!

Time of Day to Exercise

There is no ideal time of day to exercise, the only ideal is consistency; choosing a time that is convenient will make it more enjoyable and easier to stick to your program.

Benefits of Early Morning Workouts

- Early morning is the only time of day when distractions will not divert your attention from the task at hand, potentially causing you to miss your workout
- Increases mental sharpness which is a great way to start the day
- Provides energy for the rest of the day
- Regulates appetite for the day

Benefits of Afternoon or Evening Workouts

- Late afternoon is best for optimal workout performance quality
- We are physically stronger and have more endurance in the late afternoon
- Exercise is a good stress reliever at the day's end
- Evening workouts should be completed at least 60 minutes before bedtime so as to not disturb the sleep cycle. A whey protein shake is your best choice after an evening workout, as opposed to a full meal!

Studies have shown that your ability to maintain exercise intensity adapts to your chosen training time. Therefore, if you play tennis twice a week in the evening, you will enhance your game by committing to your *Body Sculpting with Kettlebells* workout on the alternate evenings. Conversely, if you are training for a morning event, choose to consistently workout in the morning.

Forget the Scale

You know that muscle weighs more than fat, so measuring your progress by the scale alone is bound to set you up for undeserved disappointment. The scale, that addictive, show-me-what-I-want-to-see 'truth-teller', actually misrepresents the facts. As you know, your weight can fluctuate from day to day depending upon hormones, health issues, water retention and sleep.

A pound is a pound, yet muscle takes up less space than fat, resulting in what should be a noticeable change in the way your clothes fit and the way you feel.

It is not unusual for a woman to weigh 5 lbs more than she did when starting the *Body Sculpting with Kettlebells* program, yet find that her pants are now two sizes smaller! This is the result of her body fat percentage shrinking, changing her entire silhouette. Remember, the more muscle you have, the higher your metabolic rate and the more fat you'll burn throughout the day and night. Rely on your clothes, measurements and how you feel as the true indicators of your progress.

Workouts by Time vs. Reps

The Strength/Endurance Challenge:
Performing timed sets with a clock provides a significantly more effective workout than one that is self-paced.

Timed sets offer more than just the development of strength endurance.

This style of workout helps you discover ease within the work. As you pace yourself with the clock, you will learn the fine art of relaxing while under tension, expending only the energy that's needed. This makes you tremendously efficient in any physical endeavor you partake in whether it be endurance for a hike, running around with children or carrying grocery bags up a few flights of stairs.

It is also an extremely effective style of training for focusing one's attention. It is simply amazing how potential distractions fade away when you're inside your 'time zone'!

Suppose I gave you an assignment: Take four minutes to perform the Swing Clean (see page 81), 30 reps on the right, 30 on the left. That may sound pretty tough. But let's consider another way of thinking of this task so that it is not at all scary, but in fact, very do-able!

The assignment is not 60 reps, simply 15 Swing Cleans per minute—not tough at all! Simply set your intention to focus on achieving four 1-minute goals as opposed to one 4-minute goal.

It is important to consider the pacing of your timed drills. You'll discover that certain movements cannot be easily paced, such as Double and Single Arm Swings (see pages 58 and 60). The objective of timed swings is to enhance overall endurance while maintaining proper form, without hastening or slowing the natural rhythm of the bell's momentum. Other exercises are easy to pace because they begin or end in a static position, such as Swing Clean and Swing Snatch (sees pages 81 and 63). The static position of these exercises is the rack and

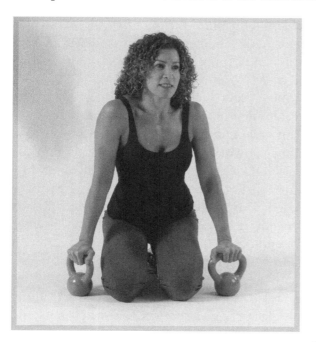

straight arm overhead, respectively. You should not perform the reps in a timed set in rapid-fire succession. If you do, you will fatigue before meeting your timed goal. Instead, relax and take a breath in the static position prior to each new rep. Each session of timed sets offers examples as to how many reps should be performed within the given time. These examples are given only on exercises that have static positions in which rest can be taken. The number of reps suggested will help you pace yourself and keep you from resting too much!

Spinal Stability

For those who have never exercised, or are returning to exercise after many months, it is very common to find the kettlebell movements to be physically challenging, particularly in performing the swing.

In these situations, the deeper (intrinsic) muscles, who are responsible for rapidly responding to changing inertia and direction, is not functioning optimally—if at all.

This motor inhibition is the result of the superficial musculature becoming the dominant 'responder'. By performing the spinal stability movements below prior to your *Body Sculpting with Kettlebells* workout, you will begin to incorporate activation of the deeper muscles, reestablishing the ability to meet the demands not only of your workout, but activities of sports and daily living.

Repeat each movement 2-3 times.

Bridge Position

1. Lie on your back with knees bent and feet flat on the floor. Tighten your abdominal muscles without pressing your low back to the floor.

Lift your butt and lower spine off the floor, so your weight is in your feet and upper spine. Hold for 10 seconds and slowly lower your hips to the floor.

2. From the bridge, alternately raise one heel at a time.

    Hold 10 seconds each side.

3. When this becomes easy, from the bridge position, raise one leg straight so that it is level with the knee of the bent leg. Keep hips even, not tilted.

    Hold for 10 seconds each side.

Quadruped Progression

1. From all fours, come into a neutral spine position so your back is completely flat. It should feel as if you could rest a teacup on your lower back.

2. Keeping your spine from shifting, lift one arm straight in front of you.

3. Return your hand to the floor and lift one leg straight behind you.

4. Once you've completed both sides, lift your opposite arm and leg. Hold for 5-10 seconds, keeping your spine from shifting.

Neutral Plank Position

1. Place your forearms on the floor, elbows in line with your shoulders. The balls of your feet should remain on the floor. Keep your abdominals tight as you hold this position for 30 seconds.

2. Place your hands on the floor, wrists in line with your shoulders. The balls of your feet should remain on the floor. Keep your abdominals tight as you hold this position for 30 seconds.

Side Plank Position

1. Place your elbow on the floor in line with your shoulder, with fingers facing in front of you. Upper leg is stacked on top of the lower leg.

2. Keep your abdominals tight and lift your hips off the floor.

3. Try to keep the upper arm resting on your upper thigh, not on the floor in front of you.

    Hold for 15 seconds.

Nutrition Guidelines

5

Getting Your Nutrition

This book offers a broad and realistic approach to nutrition without the burden of counting calories or weighing food. *The Body Sculpting with Kettlebells* workout is so effective that by following the program and making a habit of choosing nutrient-rich foods at the right time of the day, you will be on your way to feeling your best while reshaping your body.

To reiterate, consistency both in exercise and nutrition is the key to reaching and maintaining your goals. Keep in mind that regular exercise does not give you a license to eat whatever you want, whenever you want. That would defeat the whole purpose of your hard work! Understand that as your metabolism rises, you will be able to enjoy the foods you love, as long as you eat them in proper portions at the right times of the day.

You need not go on a guilt trip if you occasionally indulge in your favorite foods. Food should not be approached with the ideal of perfection or never slipping up. What matters is what you do next which is to look at your goal once again and reaffirm your intention to achieve it. Each day is a new opportunity to make choices that work in your favor. There will be days when you're too stressed to workout. There will be days when you eat junk food and there will be days when you won't get adequate sleep. The lifestyle changes you're making need to be realistic so that they are attainable as well as sustainable.

For example, if you love potato chips, it is unrealistic to imagine you will give them up permanently. But what you can do is find ways to enjoy that kind of snack on occasion, in a healthier way. Choose chips that are baked,

Consistency both in exercise and nutrition is the key to reaching and maintaining your goals.

lower in sodium and whole grain. You can also choose to save them as a reward food once or twice per week. If you have a large bag of chips, put a serving size or two into a small bowl and eat only that portion. This way of dealing with food will be satisfying and last a lifetime.

Understanding the Basics

Carbohydrates

In the past decade low-carbohydrate diets have become very popular in the pursuit of weight loss. The truth is that restricting carbs will indeed help an individual shed excess weight, but the caveat is that low-carb diets and resistance workouts do not work well together.

The most effective source of exercise energy comes from carbohydrates; therefore they should make up the largest percentage of your diet. As you will experience, kettlebell sculpt movements utilize multiple muscle groups at one time, requiring the body to have plenty of energy stores from which to draw. In addition, limiting your carb intake will leave your muscles depleted, not only of strength and endurance, but also of the firm, toned and sexy look you are striving for.

Active individuals who follow a moderate to high carbohydrate diet can maintain high intensity exercise for a longer period than those on a lower-carbohydrate diet.

Let's revisit the sports car analogy. Imagine that you are towing a heavy object attached to your automobile. Physics tells us that the heavier the load, the more force the car must provide. That force will utilize fuel in excess since it will be burned at an accelerated rate. Of course, the lighter the load, the less force and fuel required. This simple example illustrates the importance of your fuel source, carbohydrates, as you are the mover of the load.

Carbohydrates consist of two categories: simple and complex.

Simple carbohydrates are easily absorbed and provide immediate energy, making them the ideal choice prior to an early morning workout and immediately after a workout along with some protein. Good sources are fruit, juice, bread and energy drinks. Limiting consumption of simple carbs to before and just following your workout will keep your blood sugar levels steady and help reduce fat.

Complex carbohydrates provide "timed-release" energy and take longer for the body to absorb. Therefore, they should be eaten 2 to 3 hours before exercise.

Examples of energy-sustaining complex carbs are oatmeal, brown rice, sweet potatoes, grains, beans and pasta prepared al dente.

Active individuals' diets should consist of approximately 55-60% of their daily intake obtained from carbohydrates, 30% or less from fat and 15-20% from proteins.

Fats

Foods high in fat do not necessarily cause you to be fat, but overeating fat-laden foods leads to excessive calorie-intake. This is because fat, at 9 calories per gram, contains twice the caloric content of protein or carbs at 4 calories per gram. The human body gains weight only when more calories are consumed than are burned, regardless of the food choice. Fat is important for the body's delicate energy and hormonal balance, the health of the joints, as well as to make you feel more satisfied after a meal.

The basic types of fats are:

1. **Monounsaturated and polyunsaturated:** These two unsaturated fats are found mainly in fish, nuts, seeds and oils from plants, such

as salmon, trout, herring, avocados, olives, walnuts and liquid vegetable oils such as soybean, corn, safflower, canola, olive and sunflower.

Both polyunsaturated and monounsaturated fats may help lower your blood cholesterol level. Among these healthy fats, omega-3 fatty acids may be especially beneficial to your heart, as they appear to decrease the risk of coronary artery disease. They may also protect against irregular heartbeats and help lower blood pressure levels.

2. **Saturated and trans fat:** These are the less healthy kinds of fats because they can increase your risk of heart disease by increasing your total and LDL cholesterol. Saturated fat is most commonly found in foods from animals such as beef, veal, lamb, pork, lard, poultry fat, butter, cream, milk, cheeses and other dairy products made from whole milk. Plant foods high in saturated fat include coconut, palm and other tropical oils. Trans fats are made from a process called hydrogenation, which solidifies the fat, causing it to maintain a longer shelf life. Trans fats are commonly found in processed foods such as crackers, cookies and cakes as well as in fried foods. Fortunately, food manufacturers are required to list trans fat content on nutrition labels so look for them and avoid them.

Protein

Protein is essential for repairing and toning muscle, helping the reproductive and digestive systems as well as the heart and kidneys to function properly. It is necessary for the production of hormones and aids the immune system by forming antibodies to combat bacteria and viruses. Protein-rich foods provide large amounts of essential nutrients such as calcium and iron and can also help boost energy levels. As protein helps to build and tone muscle, your body raises its metabolic rate, leading to enhanced energy levels and reduction in body fat.

Lean sources of protein include grilled skinless chicken, beans, lean cuts of beef and turkey, flounder, grouper, halibut, tuna packaged in water, eggs and whey protein for shakes.

Nuts are protein rich but are also high in calories, so practice portion control.

As for cheese, use it as an accent in dishes instead of the central ingredient. Types of cheese that are naturally lower in fat include part-skim mozzarella, string cheese, farmer's cheese and goat cheese, which has fewer calories than cheese made with cow's milk.

Fiber

Incorporate fiber-rich foods into your meals such as bran, oats, barley, brown rice and the fruits and vegetables listed below.

Consuming more fiber can help you control your weight and prevent over-eating as it will make you feel more satisfied. In addition, the body absorbs fiber-rich foods slowly, which keeps blood sugar/energy levels balanced.

High Fiber Fruits	High Fiber Vegetables
Apples	Beans
Bananas	Broccoli
Berries	Brussel sprouts
Dried Fruits	Carrots
Oranges	Eggplant
Pears	Collards, Kale
Prunes	Mushrooms
	Potatoes with skin
	Sweet Potatoes
	Peas
	Peppers
	Spinach

Reduce Sugar

Avoid table sugar, replacing it with all natural Stevia or agave nectar. Choose foods and beverages that are made with 'reduced sugar', 'no sugar', and 'no added sugar' on the label. If you tend to have a sweet tooth or enjoy chocolates, cookies and cake, you may have them a couple of times a week, ideally within the Golden Hour after your workout. This is where it is important to know yourself. Can you stop after eating one piece of chocolate or three small cookies? If you know the entire box of sweets will be devoured once you've purchased it, choose to buy single-serving treats so you won't be tempted.

Be careful not to eat sugary foods throughout the day. The optimal time is in the Golden Hour after your workout.

Limit salt

Consuming more than the recommended 1 tablespoon of sodium each day will cause you to retain water, which is often very uncomfortable and counter productive. When you limit sodium your body will begin to expel more of its unwanted water weight. Be sure to read food labels and avoid or reduce foods such as bacon, canned soups, cured meats, breaded foods, full-sodium soy sauce, teriyaki sauce, chips and fast foods.

Hydration

More than 65 percent of the human body is made up of water, with nearly every function dependant upon it for the transportation of oxygen and nutrients to cells, regulation of body temperature, and lubrication and cushioning of joints and organs.

The much heralded 'eight 8 oz. glasses of water' rule is one that is tried and true, yet water does not have to be your only source of hydration. A variety of beverages and some foods like juice, milk, coffee, tea, and fruits and vegetables aid in hydration (tomatoes are 93 percent water). Recent studies show that one glass of coffee or tea provides about the same amount of fluid as a glass of water, debunking the myth that these beverages are dehydrating. The only beverages that produce a net loss of hydration are those containing alcohol.

Proper hydration is especially important during exercise since individuals can lose large amounts of fluid and become dehydrated in as little as 30 minutes. Dehydration decreases performance, impairs cardiovascular function, which can hinder physical performance, and is arguably a major cause of early fatigue during exercise.

During any form of exercise, working muscles produce heat that the body regulates by causing perspiration. If adequate amounts of fluid are not consumed, perspiration will decrease in an attempt to conserve body water. As a result, blood thickens, heart rate increases and body temperature rises, resulting in fatigue, headache, nausea, chills and possible stomach discomfort, increasing the chance of heat cramps and exhaustion. If your body is unable to cool off, you'll quickly succumb to heat stress caused by the increase in your body's core temperature.

Make it a daily habit to hydrate in the morning and throughout the day, including during and after your workout.

By the way, do not be averse to perspiration! It is wonderfully cleansing for your system and serves to cool us by maintaining healthy internal body temperature. Ninety nine percent of our perspiration is simply non-odorous water, particularly if you eat healthfully! I urge you to look in the mirror after a challenging, sweat-inducing session. You'll see that your skin glows, that it has a healthy youthful radiance! Sweating is a beautiful response to activity, enjoy it!

Limit Alcohol Consumption

Most alcoholic beverages are high in caloric content, increase hunger, dehydrate the body and slow your body's ability to metabolize carbohydrates—a process in total opposition to your goals. When choosing alcohol, enjoy a lite beer or glass of wine with a meal.

Avoid Soda

What is it about soda that is so hard to resist? It may be the caffeine, the sugar in regular soda or the artificial sweeteners in diet soda, which are addictive and tend to increase your cravings for sugars.

If you are a soda drinker, reduce your intake slowly, week by week, until you stop completely. Keep plenty of your favorite non-soda drinks on hand to make giving up this habit as easy and convenient as possible.

Although 100% fruit or vegetable juice contains many important nutrients, it also contains plenty of calories, so limit consumption to one serving a day. You may also cut excessive calories from juices by making a homemade juice spritzer. Just combine the juice with seltzer, mineral water, or club soda blends and replace soda with low calorie beverages such as iced tea, flavored waters and juice spritzers.

20-Minutes to Satisfaction

When you slow down the eating process, you will require less food to feel full. This is because the feeling of satiety doesn't really come from your stomach, but from your brain. It takes approximately 20 minutes for your body and brain to complete the communication exchange that tells you to stop eating because you're full. This process doesn't start until your stomach begins to stretch. Slowing down the pace of eating buys you time to feel full, giving you a better chance of pushing the plate away before you 'get stuffed'.

Portion Control

At restaurants, buffets or at home …

- Choose to put your food on smaller plates and use smaller utensils. This will help you to fulfill '20-minutes to Satisfaction'.
- Choose a salad as your appetizer. Lettuce is mostly water, easily digested and low in calories if dressed with a modest amount of olive oil.
- Share entrees. Some restaurants serve excessively large single serving portions. Splitting an entrée is a wise choice that you will feel good about.

If overeating is a challenge at home because you know what's sitting in your kitchen cabinet…

- Use food storage bags to pre-portion instead of grazing endlessly.
- Set a timeline that indicates when eating stops for the day—preferably three hours before bedtime.
- Do not bring home foods that you know you cannot resist.

Dining Out

Make the most nutritious and healthy choices when ordering at restaurants.

- Ask for sauces to be served on the side
- Choose light salad dressings or olive oil and have it served on the side

- Choose foods that are baked, broiled, roasted, grilled
- Choose grilled chicken or lean meat sandwiches with mustard instead of mayo
- Select broth-based soups
- Choose tomato or vegetable toppings on pasta
- Drink a glass of water and limit bread-basket offerings while waiting for your meal
- Share dessert or order fresh fruit
- Substitute a side salad or sliced tomato for french fries
- Order extra simply prepared vegetables
- Always be aware of portions
- When you feel yourself becoming full, take home the rest of your meal to enjoy the following day

When to Eat

Food is one of life's greatest pleasures, but keep in mind that its foremost purpose is to supply your system with fuel. As you create your sports car body, don't neglect it by filling it with less than premium gasoline! If you begin your sculpting session without food, you are likely to perform poorly and feel worse. On the other hand, eating too much food, or the wrong kinds of food prior to exercise can inhibit your performance and cause indigestion, sluggishness, nausea and even vomiting. The objective is to fuel your body with food that is nutritious and prevents hunger during exercise.

Carbohydrates are easily digested sources of energy whereas foods high in protein and fat will linger in the stomach for a longer time, depending how much you eat, of course. Large meals take about 4 to 6 hours to empty from the stomach. To keep your metabolism burning 24 hours, eat smaller, more frequent meals that will enable your body to process the food most efficiently, five or six small meals per day is ideal. This can be broken down into three moderate meals and two or three snacks.

Eating before exercise serves several functions:

- Fuels your entire nervous system for exercise
- Prevents hunger
- Helps prevent low blood sugar (hypoglycemia) which can cause dizziness, nausea, and headaches
- Enriches your mental state

The following food choice examples will provide your body with fuel that is easily absorbed for early mornings or up to 30 minutes before a workout:

- Banana and low-fat yogurt
- Juice and pretzels
- Sports drink
- Sports bar and water
- Fresh fruits
- Low-sodium soup and crackers
- Slice of grain bread with a teaspoon of jam

For meals 2 to 3 hours before your workout choose foods high in carbohydrates and low in fat, protein, salt, simple sugars. Good choices are:

- Whole grain cereal with sliced banana and low fat milk or juice
- Oatmeal with fruit
- Small baked potato topped with yogurt and vegetables

- Almond butter spread on grain bread with fruit
- Tuna packed in water on grain bread
- Small plate of pasta with vegetables

Eating After Exercise

It's common to neglect the post-exercise snack or meal because you may not feel hungry or don't have time, but making a habit of consuming the proper nutrients post-exercise has many benefits.

Fortunately, there is an immediate reward for all our efforts! Studies have shown that the 60 minutes following exercise is the optimal time to eat carbohydrate-rich foods and drinks. This is the Golden Hour when the muscles absorb the most nutrients and when glycogen, an energy reserve in your muscles, is replaced most efficiently. Protein is also an important component of post-exercise nutrition as it aids in recovery and helps with glycogen replacement.

Include protein in at least 10 percent of the meal. Eat a few slices of turkey on a wheat bagel, egg whites and grain bread, or a whey protein shake with fruit. Most of all, do not forget to replace fluids! Drink water, juice, carbohydrate-rich sports drinks and fruit.

Fluid, carbohydrate, and protein intake after your workout is critical. Try to avoid eating high-fat foods such as nuts or avocados in the 2 hours after your workout since they slow digestion.

As you become aware of your food choices before and after your workouts, you will experience better energy and performance levels, allowing you to reach and maintain the goals you've set for yourself. Keep in mind that good fitness habits take time and learning to eat properly is part of the process. With practice and patience, you will reap the benefits of good nutrition for exercise as well as for life.

Between Meal Snacks

Examples include: frozen fruit bars, lite ice cream, non-fat air popped popcorn, all natural cookies (no trans-fat), low-fat mozzarella cheese sticks, fresh vegetables, edamame, low-fat cottage cheese, low-fat yogurt with nuts or seeds, almond butter, whole grain crackers, apples, low-fat yogurt, nuts in moderation, baked tortilla chips.

Easy Guide

DO Differentiate between simple and complex carbs in terms of your workout and eating schedule. Always choose simple carbs if you're eating within 30 minutes of working out.

DON'T Restrict carbohydrate consumption if you're exercising consistently.

DO Eat fatty fish such as salmon, mackerel, tuna, and sardines, once or twice a week. Enjoy seeds, nuts and healthful oils in moderation.
Reduce intake of saturated fat by using lower-fat versions of dressings, spreads and dairy products, such as 1% or skim milk instead of whole milk. Trim visible fats and skins and choose extra-lean meats.

DON'T Purchase products made with 'partially hydrogenated oil' or trans fats.

DO Eat balanced meals. In order to consume the most nutrients from your food try to include complex carbohydrates, protein and a small amount of fat in each meal.

DO Eat fiber-rich foods (more than 2 hours prior to your workout)

DON'T Drink sugary sports beverages when you're not exercising. Instead, drink plain water or other calorie-free beverages.

The **Exercises**

Part III

Warm-Up Exercises

6

Key Terms for Kettlebell Moves

In order to get the most from your kettlebell workout, it is vital to understand the basic terms used to describe the exercises.

Becoming familiar with the basic terms surrounding the exercises will promote:

- Safe execution of movement
- Proper technique for maximizing power
- Proper movement patterns for creating the sculpted look you desire

Flat Back and Flexion of Hips or "Creasing"

You will see these two terms emphasized throughout the book since they are vital to proper technique and injury prevention.

Flexing at the hips means bending from the hips toward the legs. Find the front of your hip bones and place your fingertips just below them. Keep your fingers pressing while creating a crease, bringing the torso forward with soft knees.

If the result is that your butt sticks out, you're doing it correctly!

Make sure your back is flat with no rounding at the shoulders or mid-back.

Extension of Hips

Opening the angle between the hips and the legs

Example: returning to standing from hip flexion or standing up from a squat

Flexion of Spine

Bending spine forward from the waist, toward the legs

Example: rolling down

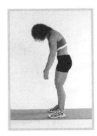

Extension of Spine

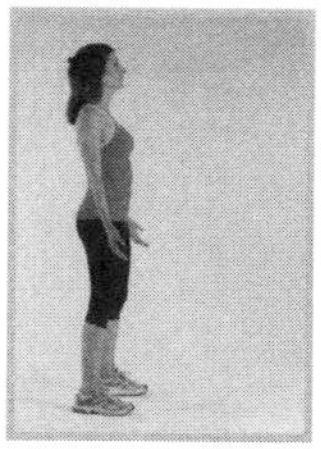

Bringing the torso away from the legs

Example: rolling up

Cross Angle of Handle

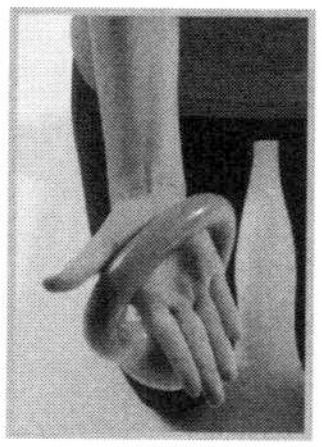

When holding the kettlebell, you want the handle on an angle with the lower aspect against the pinky side of the wrist, unless otherwise indicated.

Rack Position

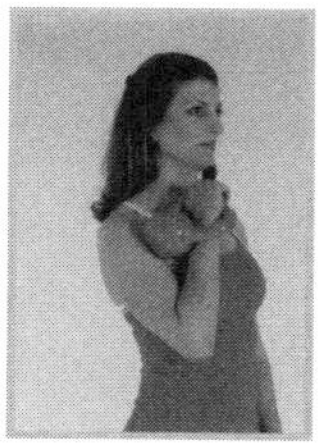

With a cross-angled handle rest the 'body' of the bell between your upper and lower arm. This should be a very comfortable position with the hand relaxed and the thumb gently in contact with the chest.

This cross-angle will enable you to keep your wrist straight in the rack and when transitioning to overhead positions.

Overhead Position

There are many exercises that begin or end with the bell in the overhead position; your objective is to maintain a straight arm and a relaxed hand.

Many people have difficulty straightening one or both of their arms fully, or one may straighten more than the other. Unless there is a preexisting injury to the shoulder or elbow joint, this is usually the result of poor movement patterns of the shoulder complex or an imbalance of the soft tissues of the arm or shoulder.

It is recommended that you see a qualified massage or ART practitioner to open these soft tissues so that you can maintain the kettlebell overhead with a straight arm. In this way the bones of the arm are properly stacked, supporting the weight instead of your muscles.

In the overhead position, relax the hand. It works hard enough throughout all the kettlebell exercises, this is one of a few positions where it can take a much-needed rest. You will notice that the straighter your arm, the more the hand can relax.

Be sure that your shoulder is pressing down whenever the arm rises up. If the shoulder complex is properly mobile, it should press down, not come along with the arm as it rises overhead.

Clean

The clean is a power move in Olympic lifting as well as kettlebell lifting. When performing the clean, you will power the kettlebell from a position below the knees to the rack. The shape of the kettlebell allows the clean to be performed in a swing or a vertical pattern.

Swings

The swing is the hallmark of the kettlebell, with its handle allowing for variable circular patterns using momentum. Swings are generated by hip flexion and extension and can be taken through many ranges of motion.

Warming Up

The warm-up is akin to performing scales prior to a concert; it is as much psychological as physical, particularly as your skills grow.

It is performed during the first few minutes of each session when your focus turns to your connection to your body and the day's workout. Do not forego the warm-up.

What are the Benefits of a Warm-Up?

- Increases heart and lung's capacity to perform during exercise
- Increases blood flow to muscle and connective tissue
- Increases oxygen exchange capacity
- Increases mental preparation
- Increases metabolic rate

Take as much time as necessary to master these movements if they prove to be challenging. You may even use the warm up as your workout before commencing the basic kettlebell exercises.

Remember, start at the appropriate level and your desired results will follow!

You will experience gradual and consistent progress if you work at levels that are appropriately challenging. Do not jump ahead if you haven't fully mastered the preliminary exercises of the warm up.

Mirror-Wiping Arm Circles

With arm straight, make large circles in front of you.

Right arm circles clock-wise, left counter-clock-wise

Perform 10 each

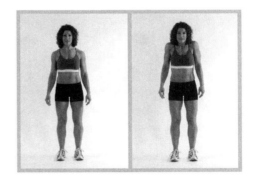

Neck Stretch: Ear to Shoulder

Stretch your neck by pressing your head down toward your shoulder.

Perform 4 each

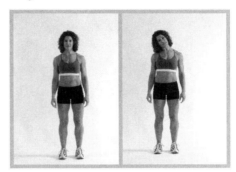

Shoulder Lifts

Raise shoulders to ears, then let them drop.

Perform 10

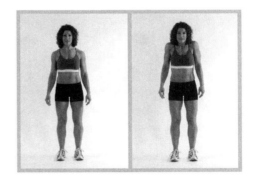

Boxer's Torso Twist

With your hands up like a boxer, keep hips stable, and rotate the spine and shoulders.

Perform 10

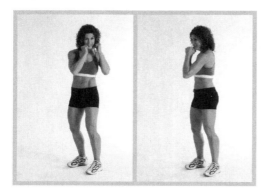

Punches

Alternate right, left, letting your spine and shoulders rotate, not just your arms. Hips and legs remain steady.

Perform 10

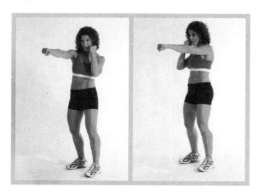

Chest Contract / Expand

With arms extended behind you, parallel to floor, press your chest out. Inhale. Bring your arms forward, reaching forward as your chest goes back, and place your chin to chest. Exhale.

Continue in a smooth manner, creating flexibility in the upper spine.

Perform 5

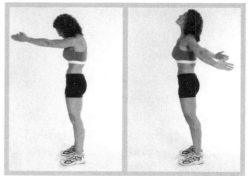

Lateral Reach Over

Reach your arm up and over your head to one side then switch arm/side. Hold each side for 5-10 seconds.

Perform 4 each

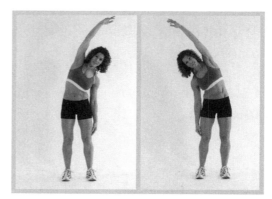

Reach Overhead, Elbows to Knee

Reach arms straight overhead, bring elbows to knee, alternating.

Perform 10

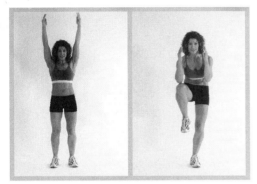

Squat

Stand with your heels directly under your hips and toes turned out slightly. Flex (crease) at your hips and send your butt back as if you're about to sit in a chair.

Keep your head in line with your spine and your eyes looking straight ahead.

Perform 10

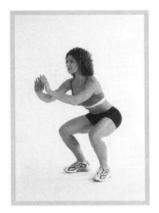

Lateral Lunge

Keep one leg straight as you lunge to the side.

Perform 5 each

Posterior Lunge

Maintain hip-width between your feet when you lunge. Make sure the front of the lunging foot is facing forward, not out to the side.

Perform 5 each

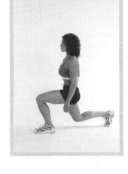

Jumping Jacks

Keep arms as straight as possible

Perform 15

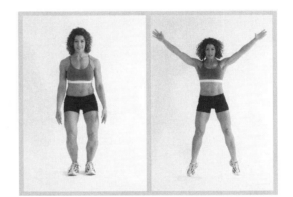

Roll Down Series

1. With knees soft, tuck your chin to your chest and on the exhale roll down.
2. Keep knees soft, arms and head relaxed, and just hang as you create length in the spine. Walk hands out, coming into the plank position, keeping your body totally straight
3. Up Dog: Pull your chest through your arms, look up.
4. Down Dog: Tip your hips up towards the sky, keep your arms straight and crease the front of your hips.
5. Walk your feet to your hands and let your head hang. Exhale as you roll up slowly, letting your head hang until it stacks on the shoulders.

Perform 2

Images should be read clock-wise.

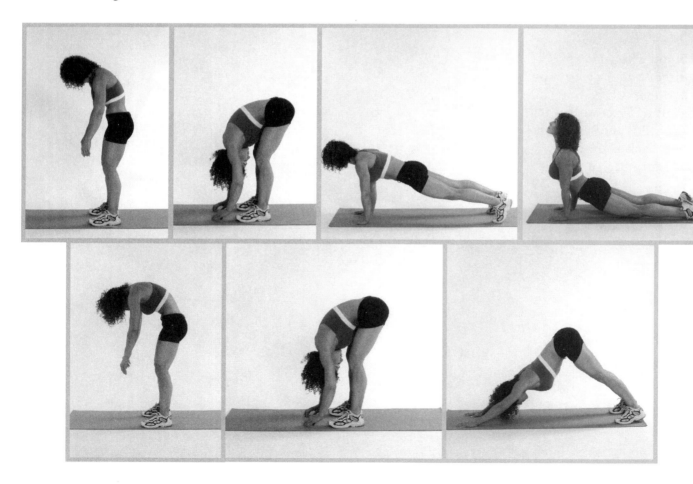

Karaokes

Moving to your left, cross your right leg in front of the left, then behind the left leg by twisting from your hips. When moving to the right, cross the left leg in front and in back. This is a coordination drill. Begin slowly, picking up the pace when it is comfortable to do so.

Perform 4 each way

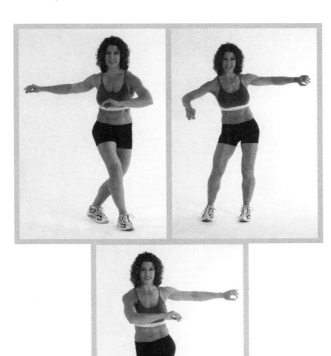

Full Body
Movements

7

Think of the exercise descriptions as recipes—read them through entirely before beginning the movements.

Taking time to learn the name of each exercise will be a great help when moving on to the Programs where combinations of exercises will be laid out.

Each of the 3 Programs are 6 weeks long, with workouts 4 days per week.

You will notice the volume of work is reduced every 4 weeks.

The purpose of this 'lighter' workload week is to give your body a break from the previous weeks' intensity, enabling you to workout, yet recover at the same time.

Taking time to learn the name of each exercise **will be a great help...**

Double Hand Hold, Squat

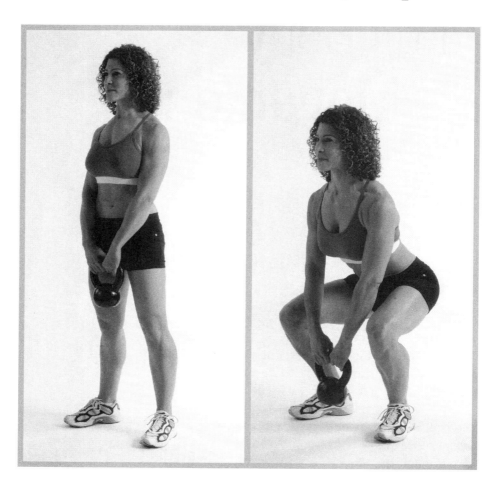

How to do

Begin with both hands on the handle, arms straight, feet under your hips, toes turned out slightly.

Flex from your hips, creasing the front of your pants as you lower your butt back and away from you, as if sitting in a chair.

Squat as deeply as your flexibility will allow, keeping heels on the ground, making sure your knees do not roll inward.

Keep your chest up and arms straight and relaxed, exhaling as you come up, inhaling as you descend.

Hanging Straight Arm Squat

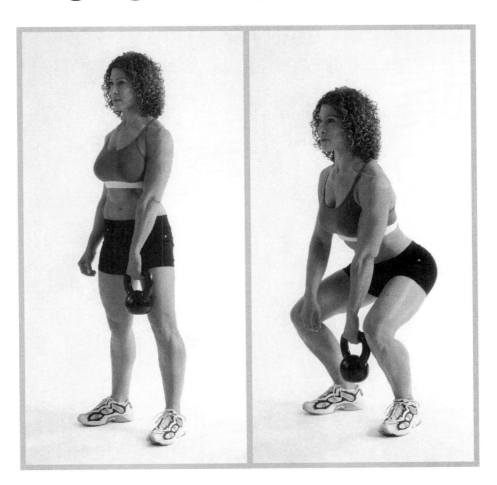

How to do

Begin with one hand on the handle, your arm straight, feet under your hips, toes turned out slightly.

Flex from your hips as you lower your butt back and away from you, as if sitting in a chair.

Squat as deeply as your flexibility will allow, keeping heels on the ground, making sure your knees do not roll inward.

Keep your chest up and arm straight and relaxed, exhaling as you come up, inhaling as you descend.

Rack Squat

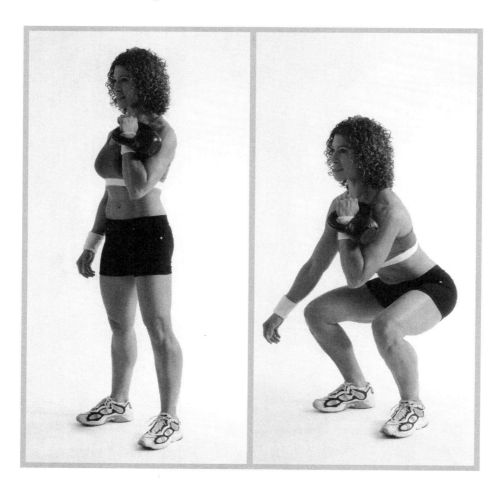

How to do

With a cross-angled handle, rest the 'body' of the bell between your upper and lower arm. Flex from your hips as you lower your butt.

Keep your chest up and your hand relaxed. The rack position should be very comfortable with no tension in the arm or hand.

Squat as deeply as your flexibility will allow, keeping heels on the ground, and making sure your knees do not roll inward. Do not rest your free hand on your thigh.

Be sure to

1. Wear wrist guards
2. Keep your hand in the middle of the handle
3. Keep your hand relaxed and in a cross-angle position

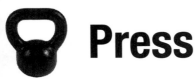 # Press

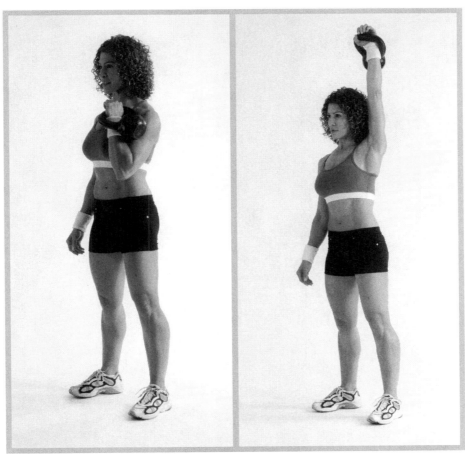

How to do

Begin with the bell in the rack position. Press your shoulder down as you unfold your arm, straightening it overhead. As your arm unfolds, your palm will face forward, hand relaxed.

Keep your legs straight the entire time and try to maintain a cross-angle of the handle.

Be sure to

1. Wear wrist guards
2. Keep your legs straight
3. Straighten your arm at top
4. Keep your hand relaxed and in a cross-angle position

Rack Squat, Press

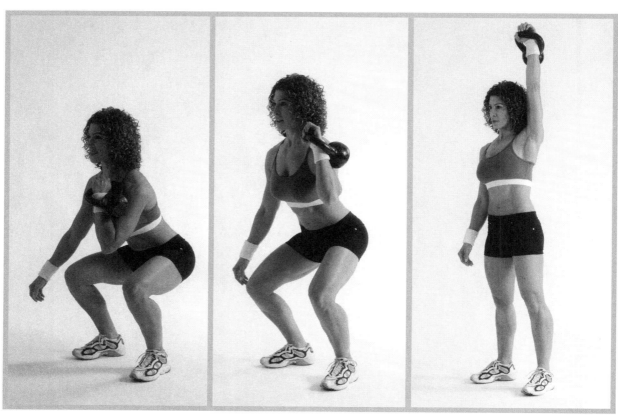

How to do

As your legs straighten from the squat, unfold your arm and press the bell overhead, straightening your arm; your shoulder will simultaneously press downward. As your arm unfolds, your palm will face forward, hand relaxed. Fold arm back to the rack and squat again.

Do not rest free hand on your thigh.

Inhale on the way down, take a long exhale on the way up.

Be sure to

1. Wear wrist guards
2. Straighten your arm at top
3. Keep your hand relaxed and in a cross-angle position

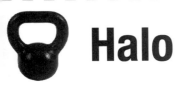

Halo

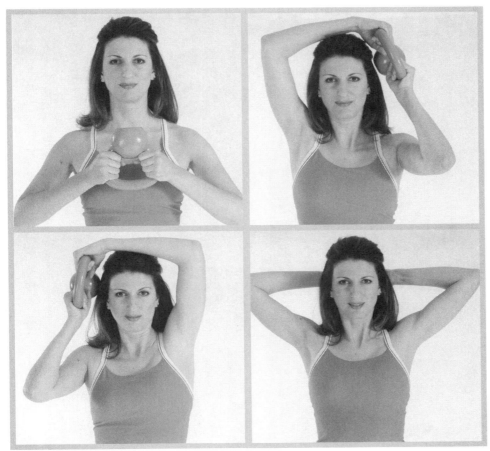

Images should be read clock-wise.

How to do

Hold bell at handles in front of your chest, bottom facing up. Starting to the left, lift the bell so it comes next to your left ear with bottom facing behind you.

Continue the circle behind your head with bottom facing down, then next to the right ear with bottom again facing behind you.

Finally, bring the bell in front of you again with bottom facing up.

Take your time with this exercise; a count of 3 seconds to complete one rotation is appropriate. Switch sides. Your forearm should trace the top and sides of your head, creating right angles at the elbow. Create a smooth and fluid movement, letting the ribcage move in opposition to the bell so that the entire core is engaged and moving.

Be sure to

1. Create a smooth, fluid motion
2. Create right angles with your forearm over your head
3. Move your ribcage in opposition to the bell

Backward Lunge, Rotate Toward Front Leg

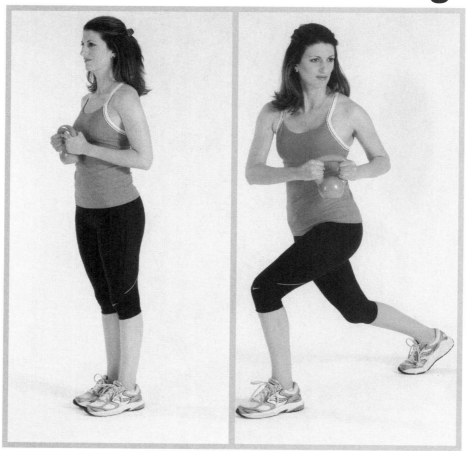

How to do

Hold bell at handles, keeping it at chest level. Step backward and descend into your lunge, then rotate your torso toward the front leg. If you're lunging the left leg back, rotate to the right to the 2 o'clock position. Lunging the right leg back, rotate to the left to the 10 o'clock position. Alternate sides.

Be sure to

1. Keep feet hip-width apart
2. Rotate your whole torso, not just the bell

Backward Lunge with Pass

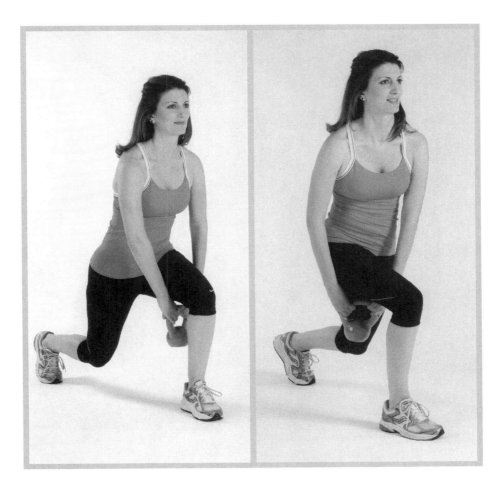

How to do

Hold the corner of the bell, lunge one leg back and pass the bell under the front leg.

Keep the space between the bell's body and handle facing forward so that you are always taking the bell at the corners.

Alternate sides.

Forward Walking Lunge with Pass

With feet hip-width apart and the bell in right hand, lunge forward with your left leg, passing the bell under the inside of that leg.

Bring back leg through, step it forward and repeat the lunge/pass.

Flex from the hips as you lunge. Keep the space between the bell's body and handle facing forward so that you are always taking the bell at the corners. Alternate sides.

Lateral Lunge, Open Arm

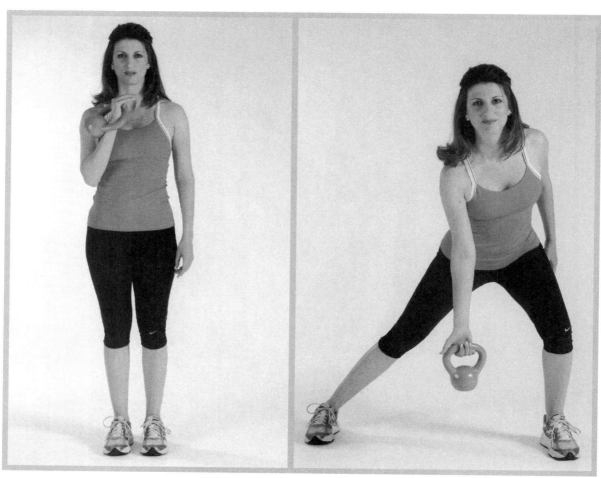

How to do

Begin with bell in the rack position. Open your opposite side leg into a lateral lunge while simultaneously opening your arm with the palm facing forward. Don't grip the handle. Instead, let it roll down to the base of your fingers, then roll back into the rack as you come out of the lunge back into a standing position.

Do not rest free hand on your thigh.

Be sure to

1. Keep the opposite leg straight when the lunging leg bends
2. Let the handle roll in palm

Lateral Lunge, Open Arm with Press

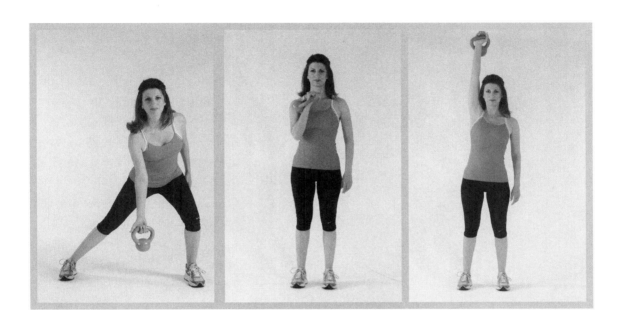

How to do

Begin with bell in the rack position. Open the opposite side leg into a lateral lunge while simultaneously opening your arm with the palm facing forward. Don't grip the handle. Instead, let it roll down to the base of your fingers, then roll back into the rack as you come out of the lunge back into a standing position. Once in a standing position, press a straight arm overhead.

Return to rack position and lunge again. Do not rest free hand on your thigh.

Be sure to

1. Keep the opposite leg straight when the lunging leg bends
2. Let the handle roll palm
3. Keep your arm straight on overhead position
4. Keep your hand relaxed overhead

The Swing

Correct Form

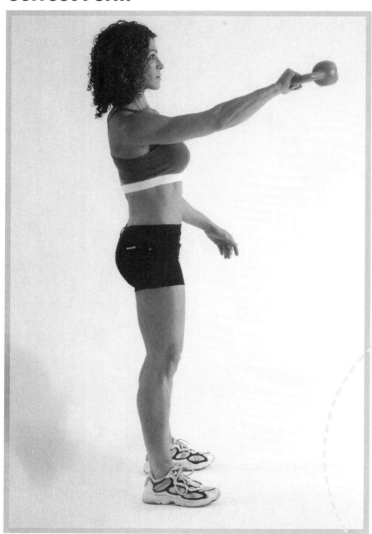

Like the plié is to ballet, the swing is the fundamental movement of the kettlebell.

A skilled swing will enable any and all subsequent movements to be guided with ease and stability.

Swings can be small or large, but will always employ the same dynamic initiation from hip flexion/extension.

Once the bell is powered up, the arm(s) will guide its path.

Be sure to retract your shoulder blades at the top of the swing to counteract the forward projection.

Incorrect Form

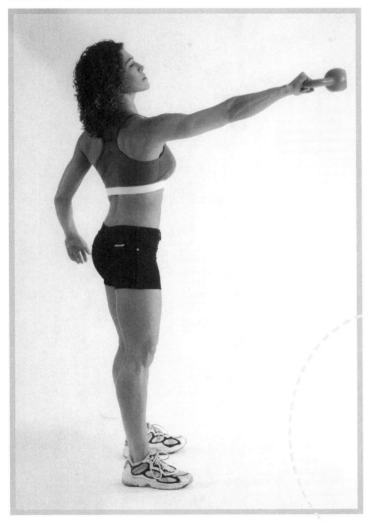

Do not let the dog pull you!

Think of the bell as an extension of your arms, which go along for the ride of the arc.

They do not inhibit the swing, nor do they dictate its speed.

Be aware!! If you become fatigued or your form starts to get sloppy, it is time to stop for the day or move onto another exercise.

Double Arm Swing

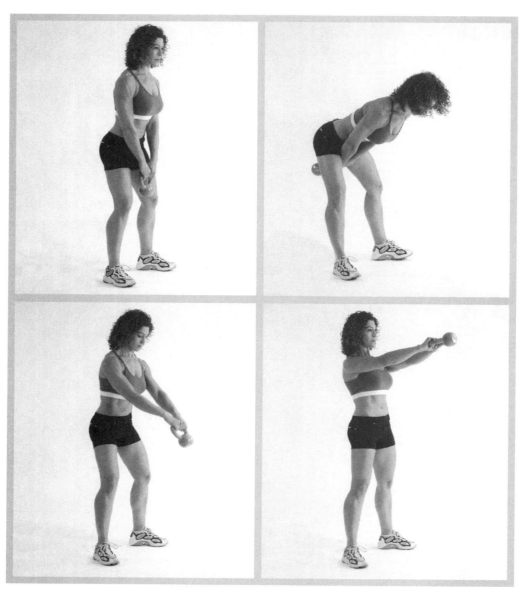

Images should be read clock-wise.

NOTE: A heavier bell such as 25 lb and above will require more effort both on the upswing and the downswing. In addition to the requisite hip flexion/extension, focus your energy into pushing your legs into the ground as you generate the upswing. This will create a very powerful force reaction, making it easier to swing the bell, while also getting you the results you desire!

How to do

Begin with hips slightly flexed, back and arms straight with the kettlebell hanging in front of you.

First, swing bell back between your legs, then use a forceful hip/knee extension to generate the forward swing up to chest level.

Keep your heels on the ground the entire time.

As the bell descends, allow it to naturally swing back between your legs, your wrists making contact with upper thighs. It is common for beginners to stop the bell short, barely letting it swing past their thighs. As you become more familiar with the swing, let it descend back as far as you can, so the entire body of the bell can be seen from a profile view. When doing this, your hips will be moving through a greater range of motion which will result in a firm and toned core, hamstrings and butt!

Let the bell fall with gravity, controlling it as it descends, not forcing or slowing its natural momentum. Arms should remain straight as the bell swings down and back between legs.

Exhale on the upswing, inhale on the downswing.

Bringing the bell to the ground: After the last upswing, take a couple of seconds to slow the momentum, letting the swings become smaller and smaller while maintaining a flat back, until the bell stops and is pointing toward the floor as in the beginning. Only then should you place it on the ground.

Do not be careless with the release! Remember, the kettlebell is still 'alive' when it's moving.

Be sure you are very comfortable with the Double Arm Swing BEFORE attempting the Single Arm Swing!

Be sure to

1. Flex and fully extend the hips and knees to power the momentum
2. Keep the bottom of the kettlebell facing away from you at the apex of the swing
3. Pull your shoulder back at the apex of the swing
4. Send the kettlebell back behind you, not down.
5. Keep your arms straight and relaxed on the downswing
6. Connect wrists to upper thighs
7. Align head with the spine when the kettlebell is swinging down

Single Arm Swing

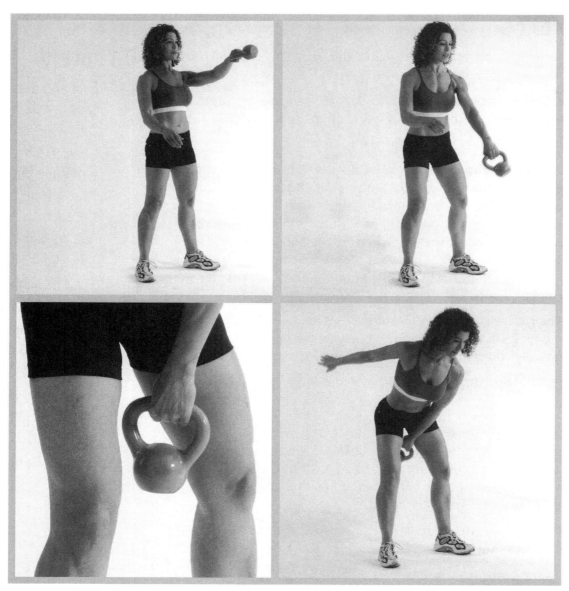

Images should be read clock-wise.

How to do

Begin with hips slightly flexed, back straight, arm straight with the kettlebell hanging in front of you.

First, swing the bell back between your legs then, use a forceful hip/knee extension to generate the swing up to chest level. Create and control a swinging arc generated by flexion/extension of hips. Once the upswing powers the bell into motion, the arm guides the path. As the bell rises, involve your upper back by retracting the shoulder blade at the apex of the swing. This will counteract the forward projection as well as protect your shoulder girdle so the bell is not a 'pulling dog' that is walking you!

On the downswing, keep your shoulder compact and steady by pressing it down as the bell goes through the legs. You should not feel as though the bell is pulling your shoulder out of its socket.

The palm will face and make contact with the same side upper thigh.

When you become familiar with the Single Arm Swing, begin to use the free arm in the same swinging pattern as the loaded arm.

Bringing the bell to the ground: After the last upswing take a couple of seconds to slow the momentum, letting the swings become smaller and smaller while maintaining a flat back, until the bell stops and is pointing toward the floor as in the beginning.

Only then should you place it on the ground. Do not be careless with the release. Remember, the kettlebell is still 'alive' when it's moving.

Be sure to

1. Flex and extend your hips and knees to power the momentum
2. Not rest your free arm on your thigh
3. Keep the bottom of the kettlebell facing away from you at the apex of the swing
4. Pull your shoulder back at the apex of the swing and down on the downswing
5. Align your head with the spine when the kettlebell is swinging down
6. Send the kettlebell back behind you, not down
7. Keep your arm straight and relaxed on downswing
8. Face the palm of the loaded hand to same side leg on downswing
9. Connect wrist and upper thigh

Single Arm Swing with Switch

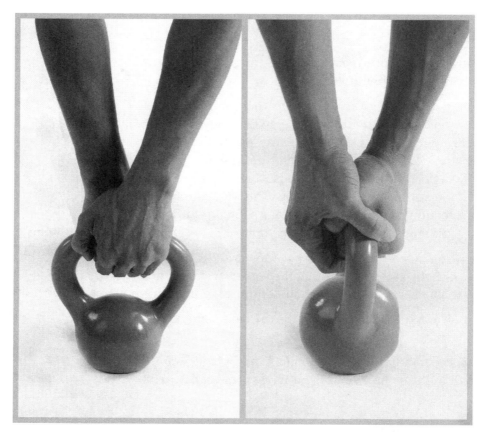

Hand over Hand **Palm to Palm**

How to do

There are two ways to change hands when performing the Single Arm Swing.

1. Hand over Hand: At the apex of the upswing, place the free hand over the kettlebell hand and switch. The change should be made quickly at the top of the swing, not as it descends.

2. Palm to Palm: At the apex of the upswing, turn both palms to face one another and switch. The change should be made quickly at the top of the swing, not as it descends. This style is a bit more challenging because it requires an additional rotation of the palm from facing the leg, (downswing) to facing the other hand on the switch.

Swing Snatch

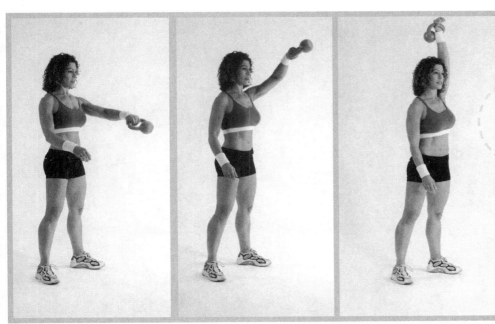

How to do

Create and control a swinging arc generated by hip and knee flexion/extension.

Gradually create a larger swing until the bell is almost straight overhead.

At the apex of the swing, relax your hand and gently punch through the handle so that the bell transitions to the back of your wrist in an overhead position.

When the timing is right, the arm will straighten just as the bell completes its transition to rest on the wrist. Relax your shoulder in the overhead position.

Bringing down: Use your whole arm, not your wrist, to gently flip the kettlebell over your hand so that it begins the downward arc.

Keep the bell in front of you at all times; it should never come close to your knee.

The loaded hand faces the same leg on the downswing. Connect the wrist to your upper thigh.

Double Arm Swing, Step-Step

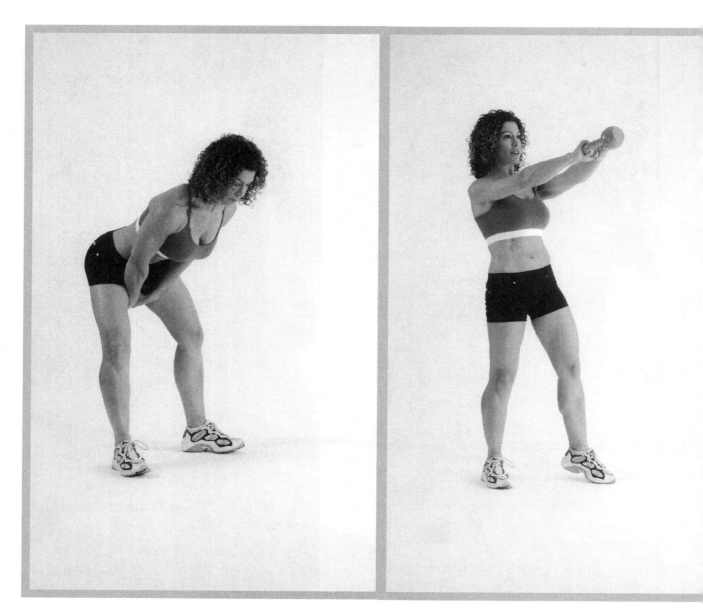

How to do

Begin with hips slightly flexed, back and arms straight with the kettlebell hanging in front of you.

First, swing the kettlebell back between your legs then, use a forceful hip/knee extension to generate the swing forward and up to chest level. Immediately after you initiate the upswing, take two steps forward, the second leg stepping parallel to the first, before the bell begins its descent. When done properly, you will be stepping just as the bell reaches its apex. This exercise is initially challenging because of its timing, but once you get it, you will have it permanently!

As the kettlebell descends, allow it to naturally swing back between your legs, your wrists making contact with upper thighs. It is common for beginners to stop the bell short, barely letting it swing past their thighs. As you become more familiar with the swing, let it descend back as far as you can, so that the entire body of the bell can be seen from a profile view. When doing this, your hips will be moving through a greater range of motion, firming and toning the hamstrings, core and butt.

Arms should remain straight as the bell swings down and back between legs.

Create and control the swinging arc generated by flexion/extension of hips, not by your back nor your arms.

Exhale on the upswing, inhale on the downswing.

Bringing the bell to the ground: After the last upswing, take a couple of seconds to slow the momentum, maintaining a flat back until the bell stops and is pointing toward the floor as in the beginning. Only then should you place it on the ground. Do not be careless with the release, remember, the kettlebell is still 'alive' when it's moving.

Be sure to

1. Hips and knees flex and fully extend to power the momentum
2. Step-step as bell reaches highest point
3. The bottom of the kettlebell faces away from you at the apex of the swing
4. Shoulders are pulled back at the apex of the swing
5. Send kettlebell back behind you, not down.
6. Arms are straight and relaxed on downswing
7. Wrists connect to upper thighs
8. Head is aligned with the spine when kettlebell swings downward

Double Arm High Pull

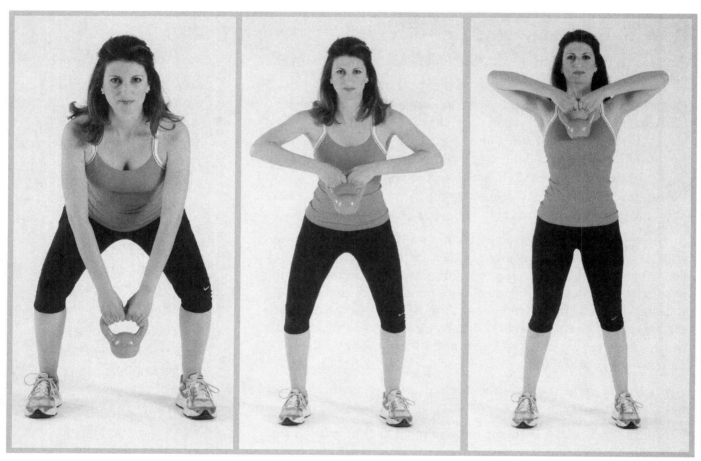

As you practice the High Pull and other power moves, you will notice the speed of your movements will increase. This power acquisition will translate into your tennis or golf game, dancing, or any activity that requires speed and power.

The high pull is a vertical power move, which means your movement intention should be explosive and fast.

This doesn't mean the reps have to be performed in quick succession, one after another. It means that when you are ready to move, move FAST, then relax, breathe and reset for the next repetition. When you are learning the movement be sure to take your time between each rep and make the movement of good quality.

How to do

As your legs straighten from the squat, unfold your arm and press the bell overhead, straightening your arm; your shoulder will simultaneously press downward. As your arm unfolds, your palm will face forward, hand relaxed. Fold arm back to the rack and squat again.

Do not rest free hand on your thigh.

Inhale on the way down, take a long exhale on the way up.

Be sure to

1. Maintain good form on each squat preparation
2. Push the floor away explosively
3. Lift shoulders and elbows high
4. Bring bell to neck level
5. Relax and prepare again between reps

Single Arm High Pull

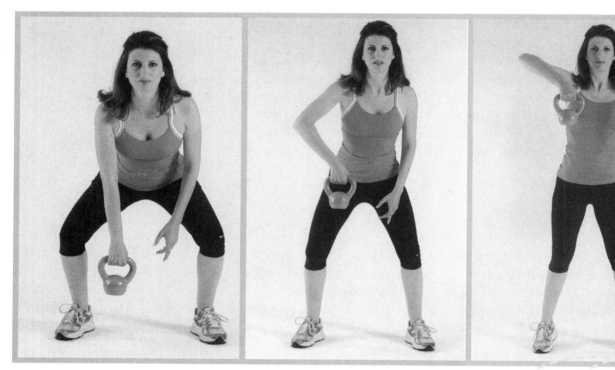

Same movement as Double Arm High Pull, but with one arm tugging as if to start a motor boat

How to do

Begin in a squat position with a flat back and with one hand on the handle, arm straight, and the bell hanging in front of you.

The initial power comes from pushing the ground away with your legs, then guiding the bell upward by lifting your shoulder and elbow up so that the bell travels in a straight line close to your body until it is neck-level. The free arm will lift to meet the bell as the loaded arm performs the High Pull, the switch of hands occurs at the apex of the pull. Keep the free arm coming up on consecutive reps otherwise you'll lose the timing of the switch!

Remember, the lower you squat in the preparation, the more power you will generate in the high pull.

Inhale in the squat position, exhale as you explode and you push your legs into the ground; shoulder and elbow lift.

Be sure to

1. Maintain good form on each squat preparation
2. Push the floor away explosively
3. Lift shoulder and elbow high
4. Lift your free arm to change hands at the apex of the pull
5. Relax and prepare again between reps

Single Arm High Pull with Switches

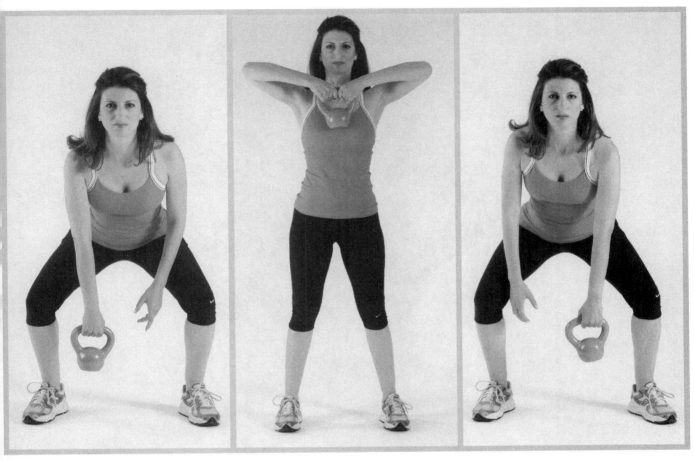

How to do

The free arm will lift to meet the bell as the loaded arm performs the High Pull. The switch of hands occurs at the apex of the pull. Keep the free arm coming up on consecutive reps otherwise you'll lose the timing of the switch!

Remember, practice makes perfect!

Inhale on squat, exhale on power of high pull.

Be sure to

1. Maintain good form on each squat preparation
2. Push the floor away explosively
3. Lift shoulders and elbows high
4. Bring bell to neck level
5. Move fast from the squat, relax and prepare again

Bent Over Row

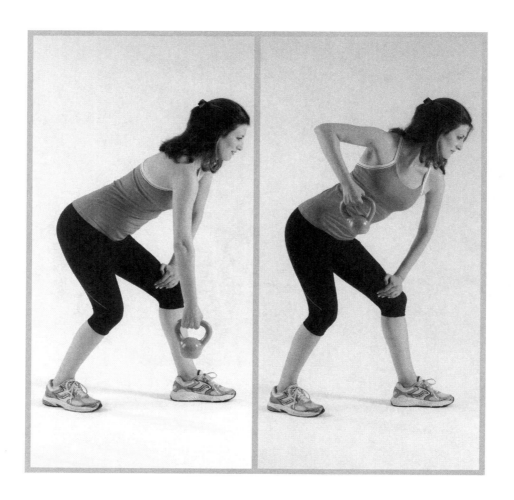

How to do

With your legs in the lunge position, pitch your upper body forward, flexing at the hips. Row the bell up to your waist, squeezing your shoulder blade back so that it's not just your arm that's pulling. Straighten your arm as the bell lowers. You can rest the other hand or forearm on your front thigh for support.

Exhale on the row, inhale as you straighten.

Be sure to

1. Bend both knees
2. Squeeze shoulder blade back as you pull
3. Straighten arm completely between reps
4. Maintain flat back

Tricep Press

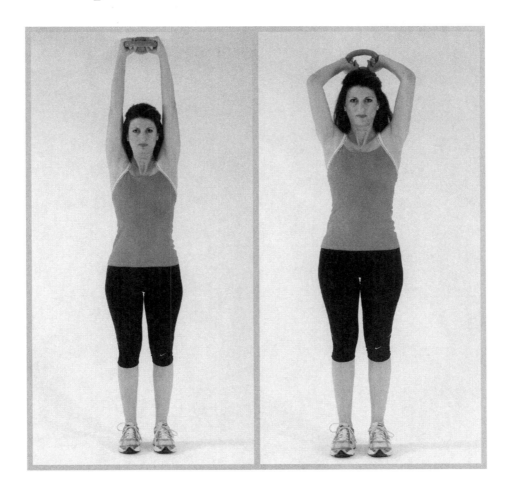

How to do

Hold handles so that bottom of the kettlebell is facing behind you. Bring bell down behind your head and press to an overhead position in a smooth manner.

Inhale as you bend, exhale as you straighten.

Be sure to

1. Keep elbows pointing forward as you bend
2. Keep head in line with spine
3. Straighten arms at the top

Tricep Press with Backward Lunge

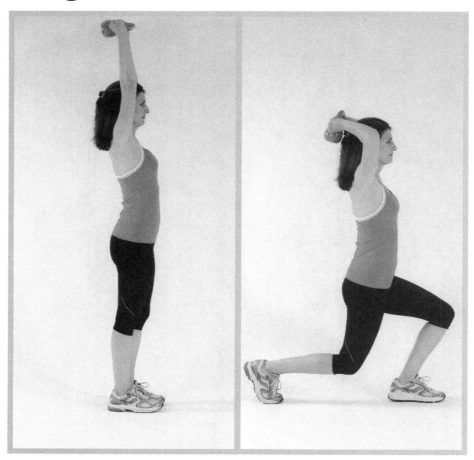

How to do

Hold handles so that bottom of the kettlebell is facing behind you. Bend your arms and bring the bell down behind your head as you lunge one leg back. Press the bell to overhead as you return to stand.

Alternate legs.

Inhale as you bend, exhale as you straighten.

Be sure to

1. Keep your elbows pointing forward as yo bend
2. Keep your head in line with spine
3. Keep your feet hip widt apart as you lunge
4. Straighten your arms a the top

Romanian Dead Lift

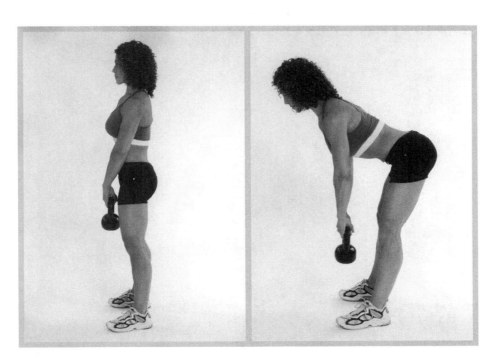

How to do

Stand with heels approximately 10 inches from a wall with legs slightly bent, heels hip-width apart, kettlebell hanging from straight arms. Flex your hips and send your butt back to touch the wall while your torso comes forward until it is parallel with the floor. Your arms will be straight, bell reaching to the floor. Return to standing.

Go as low as possible while maintaining a flat lower back. If you cannot hold a teacup on your back because it is rounding, you have gone too far.

If you feel the work in the lower back instead of your hamstrings, it is an indication that:

1. You are not sending your hips backward enough when flexing forward.

2. You are not maintaining a flat back when flexing forward.

Your head should be in line with your spine, your eyes looking forward, not down. You may stand on a stepper to create a greater range of motion. Inhale as you flex, exhale as you straighten.

Be sure to

1. Keep knees slightly bent
2. Keep arms straight
3. Have hips flex and back flat
4. Have hips move back to wall
5. Keep head is in line with spine

One Legged Dead Lift, Touch Handle

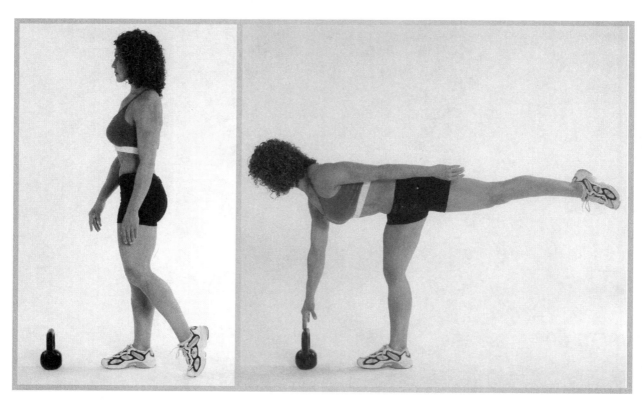

How to do

On right side, stand approximately 5 inches behind the kettlebell. Touch the toes of the left foot to the floor so that you're balancing on the right leg. Begin to bring your torso forward, flexing from your hips and bending your knee, while the left leg rises behind you. Balancing will be easier if you keep your weight toward the heel of the foot.

Touch the handle of the kettlebell and return to standing. If you begin to lose balance, touch your toes to the floor and begin again.

Keep your core engaged from start to finish and move slowly! The objective is to move smoothly with balance, not to get through the reps quickly.

Inhale as you flex, exhale as you straighten.

You may stand on a stepper to create a greater range of motion.

Be sure to

1. Flex from your hips and bend your standing knee
2. Keep your head aligned with your spine
3. Move slowly

One Legged Dead Lift with Kettlebell

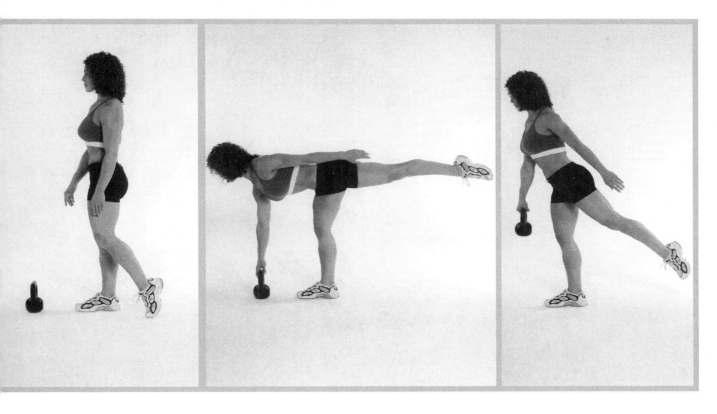

How to do

Begin with one hand on the handle, your arm straight, feet under your hips, toes turned out slightly.

Flex from your hips as you lower your butt back and away from you, as if sitting in a chair.

Squat as deeply as your flexibility will allow, keeping heels on the ground, making sure your knees do not roll inward.

Keep your chest up and arm straight and relaxed, exhaling as you come up, inhaling as you descend.

Be sure to

1. Flex from your hips and bend your standing knee
2. Keep your head aligned with your spine
3. Move slowly

Push-ups

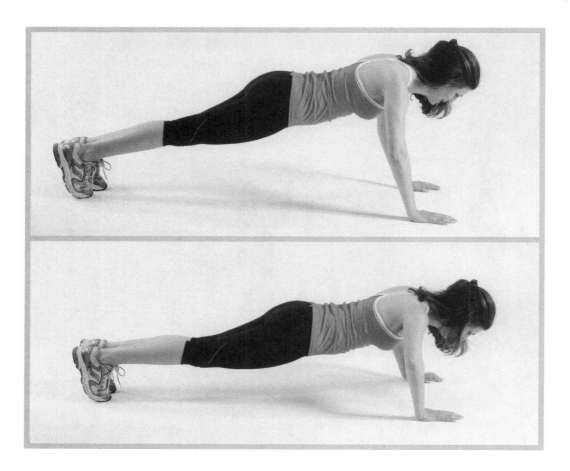

How to do

The push-up is a super core/upper body exercise that's also highly aerobic.

If you can do two push-ups with straight legs, I urge you to perform push-ups this way from here on. Try to perform push-ups with straight legs for as many reps as you can. It is okay to finish on your knees if necessary. The more push-ups you do, the easier they will become, so don't skip them!

Inhale as you descend, exhale on the push.

Be sure to

1. Keep your head aligned with your spine
2. Maintain a strong core
3. Go as deep as you can on each rep

Squat/Stand Figure 8

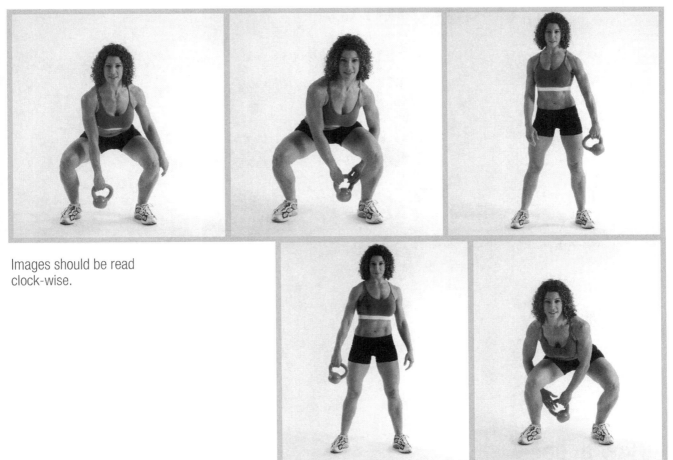

Images should be read
clock-wise.

How to do

Hold the kettlebell in the corner of the handle. Squat and pass the
kettlebell from inside the leg to behind and around, making the
pattern of an '8'. Allow your body to sway just enough to maintain
momentum side to side so your arms don't have to reach.

Keep the space between the bell's body and handle facing forward
so that you are always able to grab the corners.

One rep = one pass of the bell under right and left legs.

Be sure to

1. Flex at hips
2. Keep arms relaxed

Squat/Stand Figure 8 with Balance

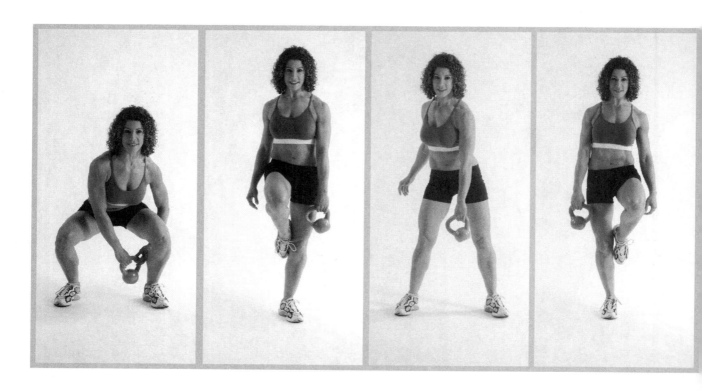

How to do

Add a balance move on each side by lifting the knee and connecting the foot to the opposite leg as the bell comes around the outside of your leg.

Balance on the same side the bell is on.

Stay in Squat Figure 8

How to do

This version of the Figure 8 challenges you to maintain your squat position while passing the bell.

Remember that shifting your body weight gently from side to side will help you pass the bell.

Overhead Press, Elbow to Knee

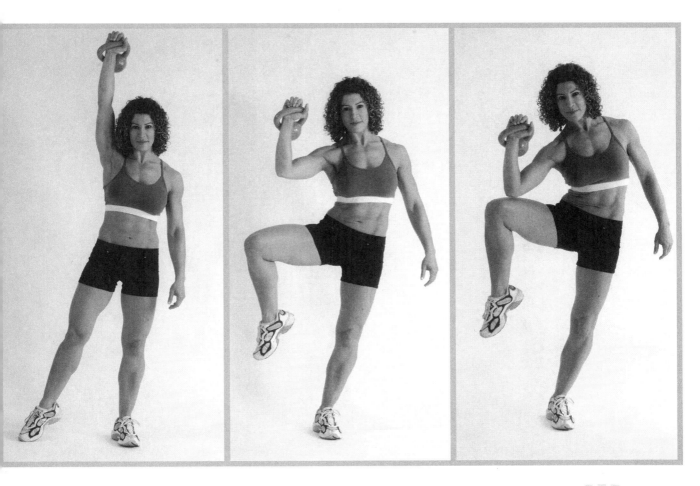

How to do

With bell in the rack position, press overhead to a straight arm position. Lower the arm so the elbow meets the lifted knee while contracting the oblique muscles. Maintain balance on the standing leg by simply touching down with the toes while pressing arm straight.

Exhale as you meet the elbow to the knee.

Be sure to

1. Wear wrist guards
2. Maintain balance on standing leg
3. Straighten arm in overhead position
4. Keep handle in a cross-angled position

Swing to Right Angle, Bottom up

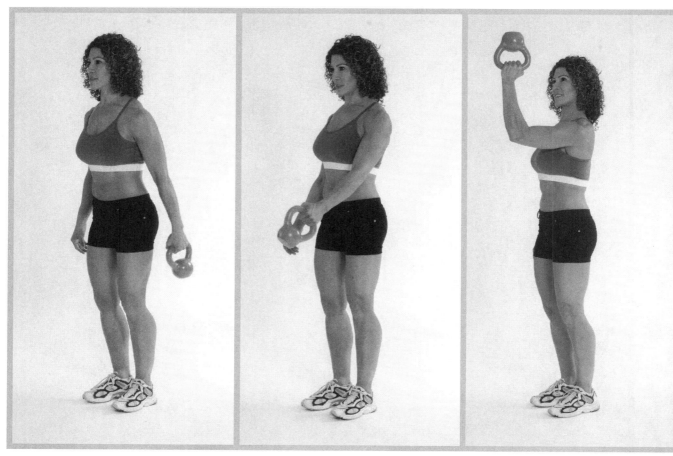

How to do

Begin with legs together, the kettlebell on the outside of your leg, thumb facing forward.

Initiate a low and gentle swing using hip flexion/extension.

On the upswing, bring the kettlebell into a bottom up position by grasping the handle, arm at a right angle. It should not look like a bicep curl and the kettlebell should be nowhere near your face. If most of your attempts result in the kettlebell flipping over your wrist rather than 'sticking' the bottom up, use a lighter bell.

Be sure to

1. Keep hands dry and lotion-free
2. Maintain low and gentle swing
3. 'Stick' bottom up, arm at right angle

Swing Clean

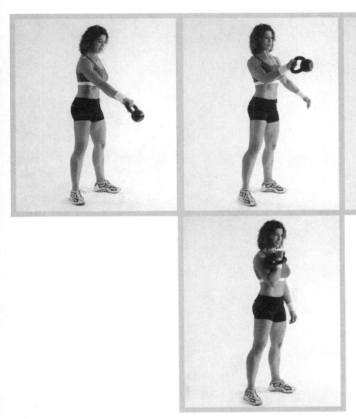

Images should be read clock-wise.

How to do

Create a low, gentle swing no higher than navel height. Then, using your shoulder and arm as guides, 'reel' the kettlebell into the rack position. Absorb the momentum of the bell by bending the knees and rotating the spine and shoulders slightly. This will prevent the bell from hitting you as it comes into the rack. Initiate the next swing by sending the bell out 45°, not down. With heavier kettlebells, you will need to accentuate your hip power and shoulder lift to guide the bell into the rack position. After the hips initiate the swing, the shoulder will lift to aid the arm as it guides the bell into the rack. Remember, this is primarily a core and lower body exercise, meaning that the movement of the bell is initiated from the hips, only then does the arm guide the bell into the rack, as opposed to pulling it in with a bicep curl.

If you can perform the swing clean with your arms alone without utilizing hips and legs, you'll want to use a heavier bell so that the use of the lower body will become necessary.

Be sure to

1. Wear wrist guards
2. Use just enough momentum to create a small swing
3. Absorb with rotation as kettlebell arrives into rack
4. Send kettlebell out gently to create next swing
5. Have palm of loaded hand face same side leg on downswing
6. Connect your wrist to the upper thigh

Push Press

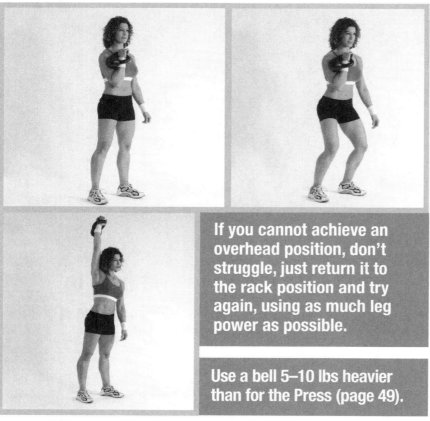

If you cannot achieve an overhead position, don't struggle, just return it to the rack position and try again, using as much leg power as possible.

Use a bell 5–10 lbs heavier than for the Press (page 49).

How to do

Begin with bell in rack position, legs straight. 'Dip' by bending your knees slightly, keeping the torso upright, then 'drive' by immediately pushing the ground away with a forceful extension of your legs. As the legs come to full extension, the arm forcefully presses the kettlebell overhead to a straight arm position. Your legs should act like a spring board that initiates the bell into motion; the arm simply guides it the overhead position.

The objective of the push press is to utilize your legs more than your arm. Use a weight that is almost impossible for you to press without use of your legs. If you can press a 20lb bell, perform the push press with a 25lb. Bend knees to absorb the weight as the kettlebell arrives into rack.Inhale prior to bending knees, forceful exhale as you power up.

Intention

As you know from the push press, your intention is to drive the bell fro the rack to overhead as quickly as possible. With all power moves, be Push Press, High Pull or Vertical Cl the intention you set prior to each is what's most important. Rememb your objective is to move the weigh fast, with power, regardless of how the bell actually moves. With time practice, your actual speed and po will meet the intention you set and will translate into all sports and dai activities.

When focusing on speed of mover most individuals make the mistake turning the entire set into an aerob class paced, rapid-fire drill. While those fast-paced rep schemes hav their place, the purpose of these power drills is not how fast you ca move consecutively, but how fast y move on each separate repetition. other words, the objective is to mo quickly to the end position, straight arm overhead, then, you're finished for that rep. You will then bring the to the starting position—the rack straight legs. Here you will reset— a breath and set your intention for next rep

Be sure to

1. Wear wrist guard
2. Use your exhale
3. Use legs like a springboard

Vertical Clean

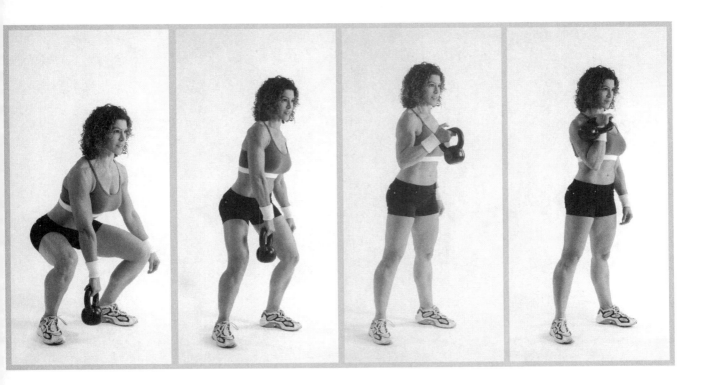

It is helpful to practice the sequence in slow motion with a light bell before putting the pieces together.

How to do

Begin in squat position, your arm straight with bell hanging in front of you. The initial power comes from forcefully pushing the ground away with your legs, then guiding the bell upward to the rack. As the bell rises, keep the palm facing your body, lift the shoulder and cut the handle so the bell rolls smoothly around the wrist and into the rack. The movement is not a bicep curl! The shoulder and arm simply guide the bell into the rack once its movement is initiated from the legs.

Cushion the bell's arrival into the rack by bending the knees.

Be sure to

1. Wear wrist guards
2. Have palm face body until it cuts under handle
3. Initiate with the legs
4. Move quickly

Two Kettlebells: One Press, One Push Press

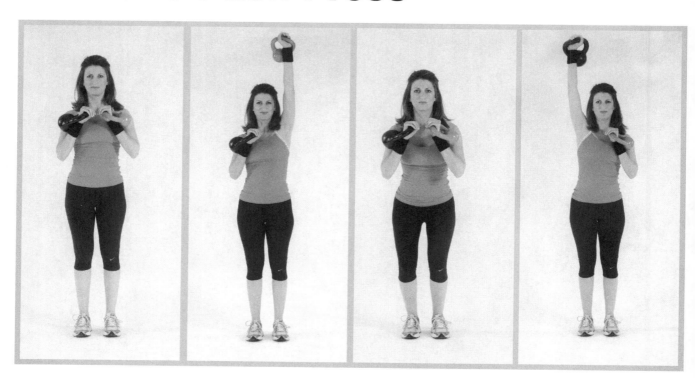

How to do

Bring two bells, a 15 and a 20lb or a 15 and 25lb, into the rack positions.

Press the lighter bell and bring it back to the rack. Then, push press the heavier bell and bring it back to the rack.

One Press + One Push Press = One rep

When reps are completed, change to the other side. Remember to use your breath to help you, especially for the push press. Inhale prior to bending knees, forceful exhale as you power up.

Be sure to

1. Wear wrist guard
2. Use breath
3. Use push press as a power move

Push Press with Vertical Clean or Swing Clean

How to do

You can add a press (overhead without using legs), or push press (overhead with use of legs) to any movement that ends in the rack position.

One Vertical Clean + One Press = 1 rep

One Swing Clean + One Press = 1 rep

After completing the Press or Push Press, bring the bell to the rack position. From here, swing it out 45° for swing clean or bring it in front of you with straight arm in preparation for vertical clean.

Windmill with No Kettlebell

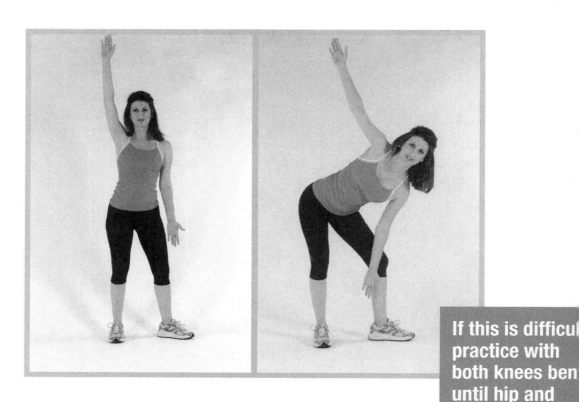

If this is difficul **practice with** **both knees ben** **until hip and** **low back gain** **flexibility.**

How to do

Smooth, graceful movement with strength.

1. No weight. Begin standing with right foot facing forward, left foot at a 45° angle with a block at the inside of the foot, right arm straight overhead.

2. Send right hip to the back corner of the room by flexing at the hips. Bend the left knee and slide the left hand down the inside of your left thigh, while your right leg remains straight. Maintaining a flat back, rotate torso, bringing your left ribcage around as much as possible. Keep your head in line with spine, and look straight ahead. Right palm will face forward during the entire movement. Touch the block with your left hand. If this is difficult, practice with both knees bent until hip and low back gain flexibility.

3. Stand, keeping your right arm straight. Change sides.

Be sure to

1. Send your hip to back corner by flexing at hips
2. Keep your overhead arr straight, palm facing forward
3. Rotate torso

Windmill with Lower Kettlebell Lift

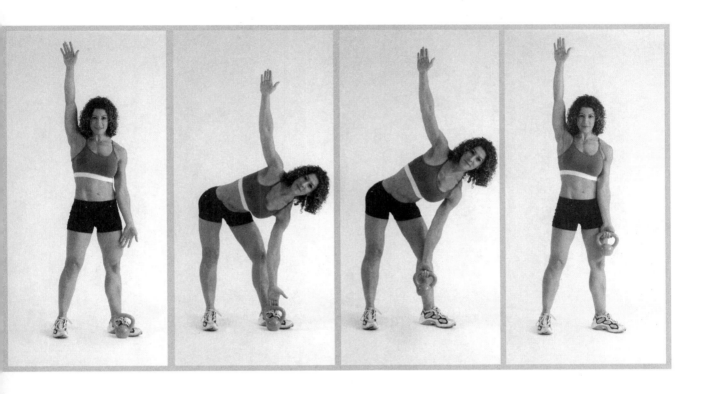

How to do

Place the 15lb kettlebell on the ground, just in front of the left foot, which will be at a 45° angle. As you flex forward, slide the left hand down the inside of your left leg and take the handle. Lift the bell as you return to a standing position. On the next descent, place the bell to the ground and stand without it. Alternate standing with and then without the lower bell, maintaining a straight right arm with right palm facing forward during the entire movement.

To make this exercise more challenging, lift the kettlebell each time you stand.

Windmill with Lower Bicep Curl

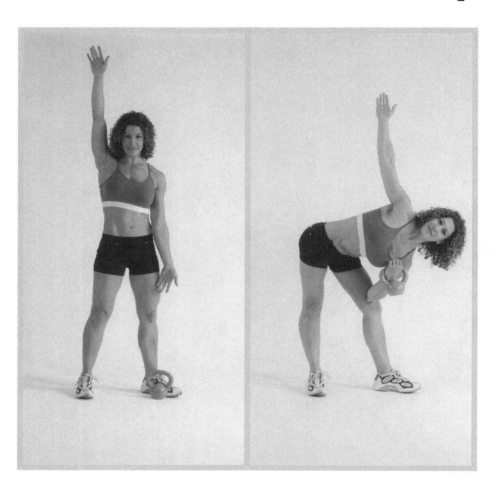

How to do

Once you're comfortable with the movement, place the 15lb kettlebell on the ground, just in front of your left foot, which will be at a 45° angle. As you flex forward, slide the left hand down the inside of your left leg and take the handle. Lift the kettlebell into a bicep curl while maintaining hip flexion, a flat back and torso rotation. Keep your head in line with your spine and look straight ahead. Place the kettlebell back on the floor and stand, maintaining a straight right arm with your right palm facing forward during the entire movement.

Windmill with Overhead Kettlebell

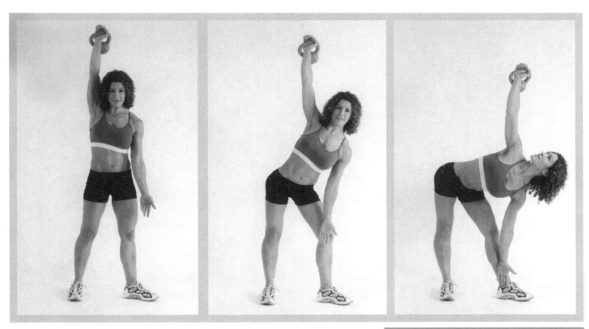

Begin with a 15lb bell.

How to do

With legs in windmill position, press the bell to a straight arm overhead. From here on focus on pressing the bell straight to the sky so your arm does not move. Instead, the body moves under your stabilized arm. You may leave your arm straight for each rep or bring it back to the rack and press it for each rep.

When you reach the Platinum Program, challenge yourself with different weights on the bottom and on the top. You can perform a set on each side with a light bell overhead and a heavier bell below. Then, on the next set change to heavier overhead and light below.

If it is comfortable, you may allow the head to rotate along with the torso so that your face and eyes are looking to the ceiling as you descend into the windmill.

Imagine 3 planes of energy -

1. From the top of your head to your hip

2. From your right hand to your left hand

3. Rotation of the entire spine, including the head

If this rotation bothers your neck or causes dizziness, keep your face and eyes looking forward.

Two Kettlebell Windmill

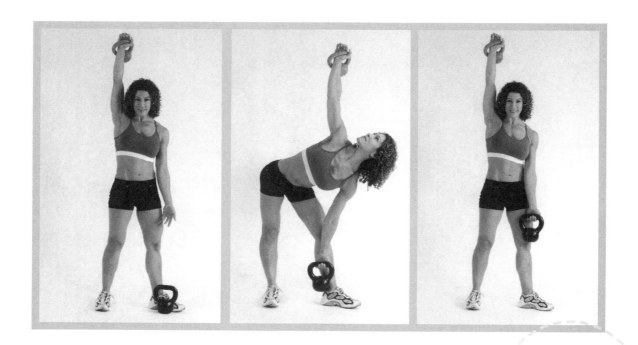

How to do

Combining the movements of the overhead kettlebell with the lower kettlebell lift.

Overhead Squat

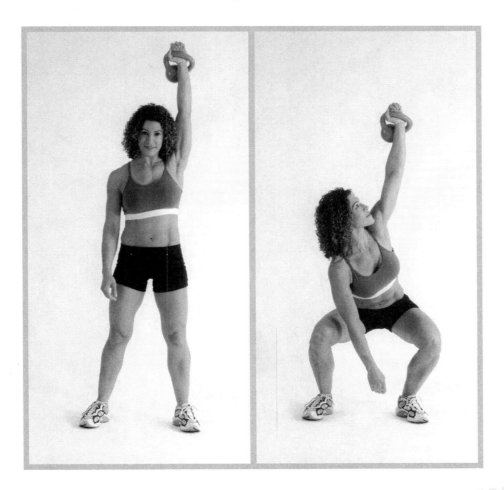

How to do

Begin standing with bell in the rack position. Press the bell overhead, keeping the shoulder down. Sit back into a squat, keeping your arm straight. You may slide the free arm inside the leg to keep your knee over your toes.

Rotate your torso, keeping your head and eyes slightly in the direction of the bell.

Return bell to the rack position upon standing. Do not rest your free hand on the thigh. Inhale as you squat, exhale as you stand.

Be sure to

1. Wear wrist guard
2. Relax your overhead hand
3. Rotate torso slightly

Super Core Strength
and Stability

8

Torso Circles

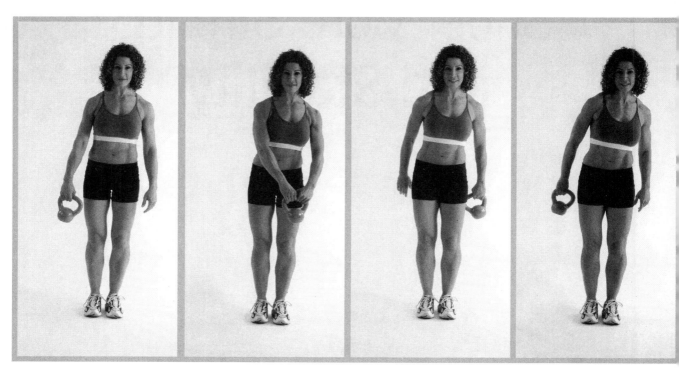

Be sure to

1. Start slowly
2. Gently sway in opposition
3. Relax your arms

How to do

Stand with feet together, arms relaxed. Slowly circle the bell around your body by passing the corners of the handle. Let your body naturally sway in opposition to the bell.

It is helpful to look at one spot in front of you, without using a mirror, this way you will acquire better awareness (proprioception) of where the bell is as it is passed.

Preparation for Turkish Get-Up

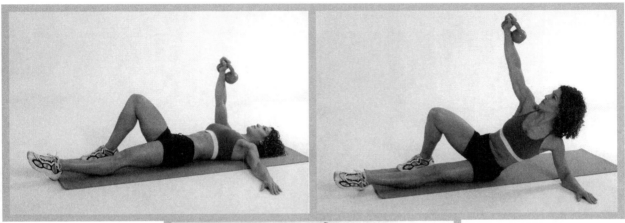

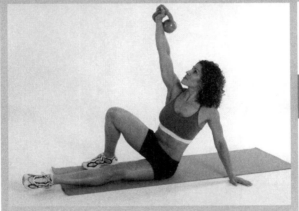

15lbs or No Weight

How to do

Begin lying on your back, right knee bent, left leg straight.

Bring the bell to the right rack position and then press it overhead.

Bring your left arm straight to the side.

Upon your exhale, push your right arm up and forward while you lean into your left forearm, then straighten your left arm as you sit up.

Return to lying as you inhale, maintaining a straight right arm, hand relaxed.

Be sure to

1. Keep kettlebell arm straight overhead
2. Lean into the free arm as you sit up

Full Turkish Get-Up

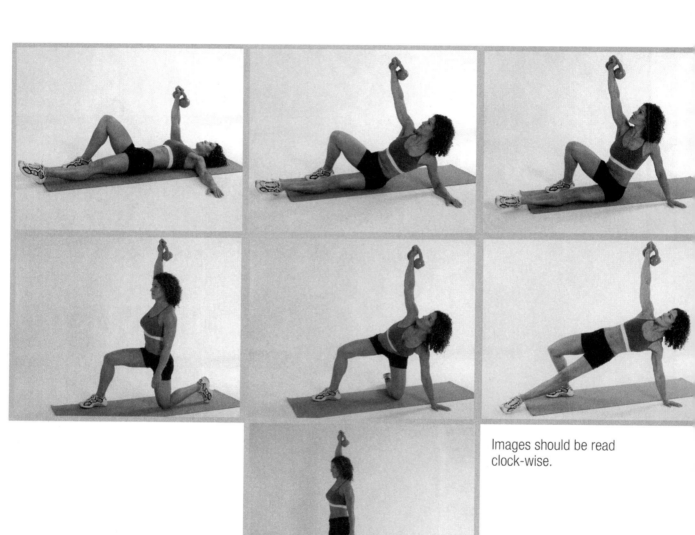

Images should be read clock-wise.

How to do

Begin lying on your back, right knee bent, left leg straight. Bring the bell to the right rack position and then press it overhead. Bring left arm straight to the side. Upon your exhale, push your right arm up and forward while you lean into your left forearm, then straighten your left arm as you sit up.

Pick your hips up off the ground, stabilizing yourself with your left arm. Bring your left leg behind the right leg, keeping your overhead arm straight the entire time.

Release your left hand from the floor and straighten out your left lower leg so that you can tuck your toes under and stand from a lunge position. Keep your arm straight the entire time.

While performing the Full Turkish Get-Up, you may use a mirror to keep your eyes on the bell as you move under it. In the first few weeks of practice you may also look up at the bell for reassurance. As you become adept at overhead exercises such as this, your skills will be better served by feeling the placement of the bell rather than looking at it, letting your body, rather than your eyes inform you.

After performing the Full Turkish Get-Up for a few weeks, wean yourself away from the mirror and 'eyes on the bell' to so that your body is a highly responsive system. After all, the more we can anticipate and respond to stimulus around us, the better we function, both in sport and in life.

To return to the floor:

Step your left leg back into a lunge, bringing your left knee to the ground. Place your left hand down for support while lifting your hips, then bring the left leg to the front and lie down. Your right leg remains bent and your right arm remains straight.

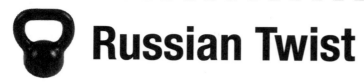 # Russian Twist

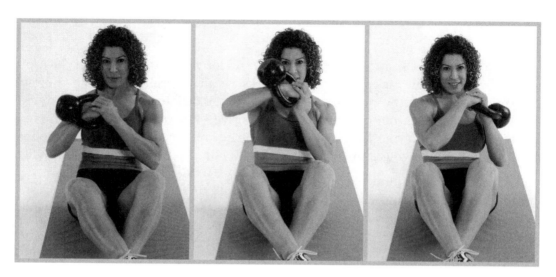

How to do

Sit on the floor with knees bent, feet on the floor. With hands layered in the handle and fingers facing one another, bring the bell to the rack position.

Lean back and flip the bell to the opposite rack position. Rotate your shoulders and torso to absorb the bell as it reaches the rack each time, maintaining a continuous pace so the bottom of the bell is always facing away from you, not down.

For a greater challenge, cross your ankles and elevate your feet for the duration of the exercise.

Flipping bell to right and left sides = 1 rep

Russian Twist Holding Handles

How to Do: Sit on floor, with knees bent and feet on floor. Hold bell's handles and lean back. Bring the bell to the outside of your waistline and touch it to the ground, alternating sides. As you progress with this exercise, try to move faster, maintaining a strong core as you move.

one rep = twist of bell to right and left sides

Be sure to

1. Wear wrist guard
2. Rotate shoulders and torso

Overhead/Chest/Sit-Up/Press

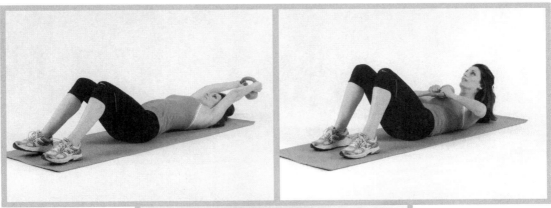

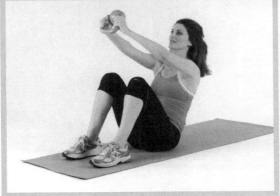

How to do

Begin by lying on your back, legs bent, feet on the floor. Hold the bell by the handles at your chest. The bottom of the bell can either face away from you or toward you. Bring the bell behind your head only as far as you can while keeping your arms straight. Create a long exhale as you bring the bell to the chest and quickly sit up, pressing your arms straight, pointing the bell to the corner of the ceiling. On a long inhale, bring the bell back to your chest and lower yourself to the ground.

If you cannot extend your arms to touch the floor overhead, use a block to dictate the range of motion that is comfortable for you.

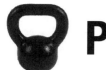 # Plank Row, Pass

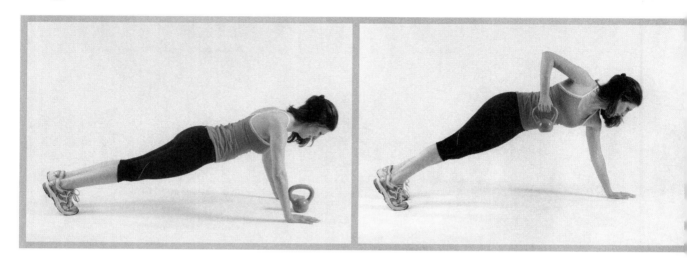

How to do

Begin in the plank position with the bell on the inside of your right hand. Row it to your waistline, stabilizing yourself through your core and left arm. Pass the bell to the inside of the left hand and row, alternating sides.

Rowing on right and left sides = 1 rep

Side Plank Row, Pass

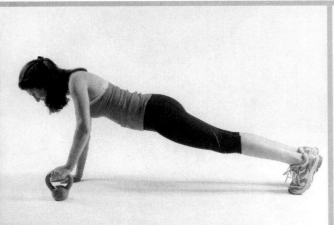 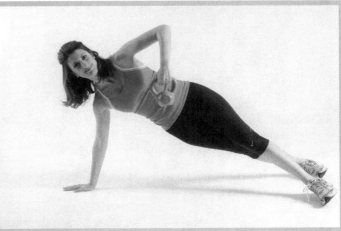

Be sure to

1. Roll to the edges of your feet
2. Keep your shoulder over your wrist

How to do

Begin in the plank position, feet open about 10 inches, with the bell on the inside of your right hand. Roll to side plank so that you are supported on the sides of your feet and your left hand with a straight arm. Your shoulder must be directly over your wrist in order for you to create a stable and comfortable position. Keep your hips high off the ground as you row the bell to your waistline. You may let the bell touch your body as you row.

Return to center plank, passing the bell to the inside of the left hand, alternating sides.

Rowing on right and left sides = 1 rep

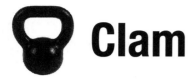 # Clam

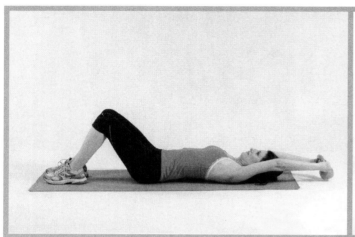 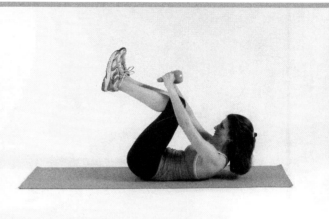

How to do

Begin lying on your back with knees bent, and feet on the floor.

Hold the bell by the handles. The bottom of the bell can either face away from you or toward you. Bring the bell behind your head only as far as you can while keeping your arms straight. In one motion, bring the bell to gently meet your shins as knees lift toward your chest.

Sit up as far as possible with your chest and head. Keep your arms straight for the entire exercise. Inhale as you lie back, exhale as you sit up.

If you cannot extend your arms to touch the floor overhead, use a block to dictate the range of motion that is comfortable for you.

Active Recovery
and Stretching

9

Active Recovery: Keep Moving Once Your Heart Rate is High

If you simply stand, sit or lie down while your heart rate is still elevated following a challenging set, you will cause your heart to work unreasonably hard to recover oxygen, potentially causing dizziness or nausea. Walk around or march in place between exercises as opposed to sitting or standing still. After completing your workout, engage in active recovery for 2 to 3 minutes until your heart rate and breathing are almost down to normal.

Active recovery is part of the cool down and includes low intensity exercise with the purpose of gradually slowing the pace and exertion of your activity.

Examples of active recovery include:
1. Torso circles with bell
2. Jumping jacks
3. Jogging in place
4. Jump rope in place
5. Backward lunges, no weight
6. Walking
7. Marching

Benefits of Active Recovery
- Allows heart rate and breathing to return to its resting rate
- Relaxes muscles and helps them return to resting length
- Reduces possible muscle spasm or cramping
- Removes waste by-products from the blood
- Reduces the chances of dizziness
- Reduces the level of adrenaline in the blood

Stretches

Stretching is best performed immediately following active recovery when the body's temperature is higher than normal. Though studies have shown that post-exercise stretching does not prevent muscle soreness, it can increase joint range of motion, increase flexibility and decrease stiffness.

Stretches should be held for an average of 30 seconds, allowing the muscles to relax and lengthen. Continue to tune in to your body when in the final stage of your workout. Use proper form and keep mental chatter to a minimum.

Be sure to stretch both sides evenly and give extra time to any areas that are stiff, using your exhale to settle into the stretch without

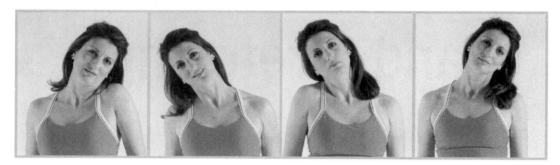

forcing.

Shoulder and Neck

Meet your right ear to your right shoulder by tilting your head and lifting the shoulder. Stretch by tilting your head to the left and lowering your shoulder, reaching to the floor with a flexed palm.

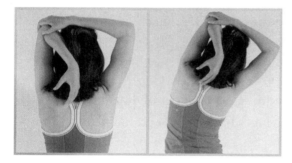

Triceps with Tilt

Place your left fingertips on your left shoulder blade, place your right hand on your left elbow and gently guide the elbow straight back. Keep your head up. Tilt your shoulders and head to the right to elongate the triceps and shoulder muscles.

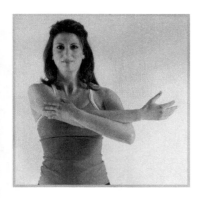

Posterior Shoulder

Bring your arm across your chest, gently holding it with your opposite hand; keep shoulder down.

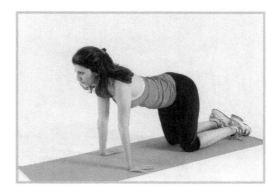

Forearm Stretch in Plank

On all fours, place hands so that your fingertips face your knees. For a deeper stretch, try to bend your elbows.

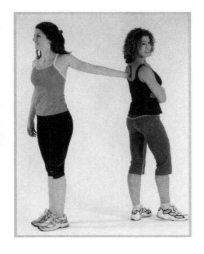

Bicep/Forearm Stretch on Wall

With arm at shoulder level, place your palm on a wall with fingers pointed behind you. Squeeze your shoulder blade back while turning away from the palm. You should feel a long stretch through the chest, biceps, forearm and hand.

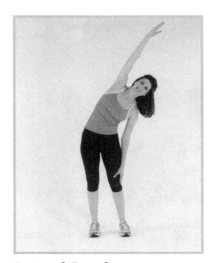

Lateral Reach

Reach your arm up and over while supporting yourself with the opposite hand on your out thigh. Keep both sides of your ribcage long, do not sink into the position.

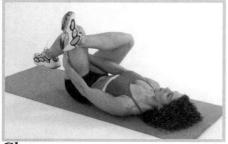

Glutes

Lying on your back, cross your right ankle over your left knee and draw the left leg toward your chest, or you may place the left foot on a wall and give your arms a rest. Dorsiflex both feet and press your tailbone into the floor, flexing from your hips.

Imagine elongating your head and hips away from each other.

Hamstrings

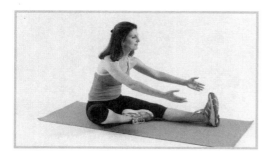

Sit with your left leg in front of you and right leg bent to your side, keeping hip bones on the ground.

Flex and internally rotate the left foot while pressing the back of the knee into the floor. Maintaining a flat spine, reach your arms forward and to the ground, lean forward as much as possible. Relax and breathe.

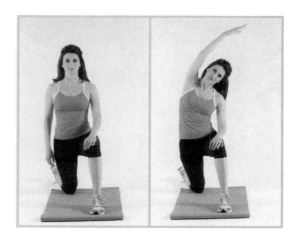

Psoas

Begin in a lunge position with your right knee on the ground, shin slightly outside the midline of the thigh.. The left leg will be slightly outside of the midline of the hip. The hips should remain facing forward and level, not tilted.

Keep your lower abdominals engaged and if possible, lunge forward a bit more while maintaining alignment of the hips.

Reach your right arm up and over to the left.

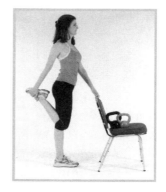

Quadriceps

Stand facing an object or wall that you can lightly hold for balance. Bring your right heel behind you, holding your foot or ankle with your right hand. Contact your right glute as you pull your heel closer to your butt.

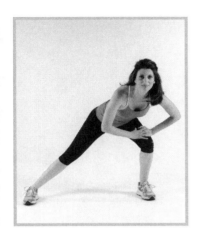

Inner Thighs

With legs wide and feet parallel, lunge deeply into the left leg, keeping your right leg straight. Lean your hands onto the floor or your thigh, keeping your low back flat as you flex from your hips. As you bend into the left leg, press the right foot down into the floor and away from you.

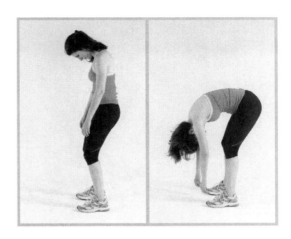

Roll Down/Up

With legs hip width apart and knees slightly bent, tuck you chin and roll down slowly as you exhale. Your head and arms hang relaxed until you reach the end of your range of motion. Hang for 20-30 seconds breathing deeply and gently shaking your head as if saying 'no' and 'yes' to release your neck muscles. You may keep your legs bent for this spinal stretch. On an exhale, slowly roll up, stacking one vertebra at a time with shoulders and head last to come upright

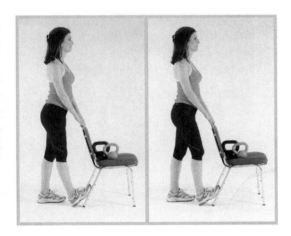

Calf

Flex your foot and place your heel as close to the wall as possible, then gently straighten your leg. As you stretch, gently alternate bending and straightening the stretching leg a few of times to lengthen both the gastrocnemius and the Achilles tendon.

The **Kettlebell Athlete**

Silver Medal Program

10

Program Level: 1
Program Length: 6 weeks, 4 workouts per week.
Weight: 15 lb and 20 lb kettlebells
Workout Length: Approximately 45-60 minutes.

Perform the exercises in order, with the given rest periods. The fourth day of each week (super-set day) is a shorter, more intense workout.

SILVER PROGRAM, Week 1, Monday				
	Exercise	Page #	Weight	No. of Reps
Warm-up				
Drill 1				
Rest Period: 30 seconds to 1 minute between exercises			No. of sets: 3	
	Double Hand Hold, Squat	46	15	12
	Halo	51	15	5 each
	Backward Lunge, Rotate Toward Front Leg (hold kettlebell at chest)	52	15	10 each
	Double Arm Swing	58	15	10
Drill 2				
Rest Period: n/a			No. of sets: 1	
	Hold Plank Position	100	n/a	30 seconds
Cool Down/Stretch				

SILVER PROGRAM, Week 1, Wednesday				
	Exercise	Page #	Weight	No. of Reps
Warm-up				
Drill 1				
Rest Period: 30 seconds to 1 minute between exercises				No. of sets: 3
	Rack Squat	48	15	8 each
	Bent Over Row	70	15	10 each
	Tricep Press	71	15	15
	Double Arm High Pull	66	15	10
Drill 2				
Rest Period: 30 seconds to 1 minute between exercises				No. of sets: 2
	Russian Twist (feet on floor, knees bent)	98	15	10
Cool Down/Stretch				

	Exercise	Page #	Weight	No. of Reps
SILVER PROGRAM, Week 1, Friday				
Warm-up				
Drill 1				
Rest Period: 30 seconds to 1 minute between exercises				No. of sets: 3
	Double Hand Hold, Squat	46	20	8
	Torso Circles	94	20	8 each
	Romanian Dead Lift	73	20	10
	Squat/Stand Figure 8	77	20	5
Drill 2				
Rest Period: n/a				No. of sets: 1
	Plank Row, Pass	100	15	6
Cool Down/Stretch				

SILVER PROGRAM, Week 1, Saturday				
	Exercise	**Page #**	**Weight**	**No. of Reps**
Warm-up				
Drill 1				
Rest Period: up to 45 seconds between drills				No. of sets: 1
	Double Arm Swing	58	20	15
	Jumping Jacks	42	n/a	15
Drill 2				
Rest Period: up to 45 seconds between drills				No. of sets: 1
	Double Arm Swing	58	20	12
	Jumping Jacks	42	n/a	12
Drill 3				
Rest Period: up to 45 seconds between drills				No. of sets: 1
	Double Arm Swing	58	20	10

SILVER PROGRAM, Week 1, Saturday				
	Exercise	**Page #**	**Weight**	**No. of Reps**
	Jumping Jacks	42	n/a	10

Drill 4				
Rest Period: n/a				No. of sets: 1
	Double Arm Swing	58	20	8
	Jumping Jacks	42	n/a	8
Cool Down/Stretch				

SILVER PROGRAM, Week 2, Monday				
	Exercise	**Page #**	**Weight**	**No. of Reps**
Warm-up				

Drill 1				
Rest Period: 30 to 45 seconds between exercises				No. of sets: 3
	Rack Squat, Press	50	15	5 each
	Halo	51	15	6 each

SILVER PROGRAM, Week 2, Monday

	Exercise	Page #	Weight	No. of Reps
	Double Arm Swing	58	15	15
	Backward Lunge, Rotate to Front Leg	52	15	8 each
	Bent Over Row	70	15	12 each

Drill 2
Rest Period: 30 seconds   No. of sets: 2

	Exercise	Page #	Weight	No. of Reps
	Russian Twist (feet on floor, knees bent)	98	15	15

Cool Down/Stretch

SILVER PROGRAM, Week 2, Wednesday

	Exercise	Page #	Weight	No. of Reps

Warm-up

Drill 1
Rest Period: 30 seconds to 1 minute between exercises   No. of sets: 3

	Exercise	Page #	Weight	No. of Reps
	Double Hand Hold, Squat	46	20	8

SILVER PROGRAM, Week 2, Wednesday				
	Exercise	**Page #**	**Weight**	**No. of Reps**
	Vertical Clean	83	20	5 each

Drill 2
Rest Period: 30 seconds to 1 minutes between exercises — No. of sets: 3

	Romanian Dead Lift	73	20	10
	Torso Circles	94	20	10 each

Drill 3
Rest Period: 30 seconds to 1 minutes between exercises — No. of sets: 2

	Plank Row, Pass	100	15	6
	Overhead/Chest/Sit up/ Press	99	15	10

Cool Down/Stretch

SILVER PROGRAM, Week 2, Friday				
	Exercise	**Page #**	**Weight**	**No. of Reps**
Warm-up				
Drill 1				
Rest Period: 30 seconds to 1 minute between exercises			No. of sets: 3	
	Rack Squat	48	15	10 each
	Overhead Press, Elbow to Knee	79	15	10 each
	Backward Lunge with Pass (alternating)	53	15	8 each
	Double Arm Swing	58	15	20
	Push-up (on knees if necessary)	76	n/a	5
	Overhead/Chest/Situp/Press	99	15	15
Cool Down/Stretch				

	Exercise	Page #	Weight	No. of Reps
SILVER PROGRAM, Week 2, Saturday				
Warm-up				
Drill 1				
Rest Period: up to 1 minute between drills				No. of sets: 1
	Squat/Stand Figure 8	77	20	10
	Jumping Jacks	42	n/a	20
Drill 2				
Rest Period: up to 45 seconds between drills				No. of sets: 1
	Squat/Stand Figure 8	77	20	8
	Jumping Jacks	42	n/a	15
Drill 3				
Rest Period: up to 45 seconds between drills				No. of sets: 1
	Squat/Stand Figure 8	77	20	6

SILVER PROGRAM, Week 2, Saturday

	Exercise	Page #	Weight	No. of Reps
	Jumping Jacks	42	n/a	10

Drill 4
Rest Period: n/a   No. of sets: 1

	Exercise	Page #	Weight	No. of Reps
	Russian Twist (feet on floor, knees bent)	98	20	10
	Plank Row, Pass	100	20	8

Cool Down/Stretch

SILVER PROGRAM, Week 3, Monday

	Exercise	Page #	Weight	No. of Reps

Warm-up

Drill 1
Rest Period: 30 to 45 seconds between exercises   No. of sets: 3

	Exercise	Page #	Weight	No. of Reps
	Rack Squat, Press	50	15	8 each
	Halo	51	15	8 each

SILVER PROGRAM, Week 3, Monday				
	Exercise	Page #	Weight	No. of Reps
	Double Arm Swing	58	15	15
Drill 2 Rest Period: 30 to 45 seconds between exercises				No. of sets: 3
	Lateral Lunge, Open Arm	54	15	8 each
	Bent Over Row	70	15	15 each
	Tricep Press with Balance	71	15	8 each leg
Drill 3 Rest Period: 30 to 45 seconds between exercises				No. of sets: 2
	Russian Twist (feet crossed and elevated)	98	15	15
	Overhead/Chest/Sit Up/ Press	99	15	15 each
Cool Down/Stretch				

SILVER PROGRAM, Week 3, Wednesday				
	Exercise	**Page #**	**Weight**	**No. of Reps**
Warm-up				
Drill 1 Rest Period: 30 to 45 seconds between exercises				No. of sets: 3
	Rack Squat	48	15	15 each
	Overhead Press, Elbow to Knee	79	15	12 each
	Backward Lunge with Pass	53	15	10 each
	Turkish Get Up Prep	95	15	4 each
	Clam	102	15	15
Cool Down/Stretch				

SILVER PROGRAM, Week 3, Friday				
	Exercise	**Page #**	**Weight**	**No. of Reps**
Warm-up				
Drill 1 Rest Period: 30 to 45 seconds between exercises				No. of sets: 3
	Press	49	15	10 each
	Double Arm Swing	58	15	15
	Swing to Right Angle, Bottom Up	80	15	10 each
Drill 2 Rest Period: 30 to 45 seconds between exercises				No. of sets: 3
	Bent Over Row	70	15	15 each
	Push-up (straight legs)	76	n/a	5, 3, 3
	Vertical Clean	83	15	15 each

SILVER PROGRAM, Week 3, Friday				
	Exercise	**Page #**	**Weight**	**No. of Reps**
Drill 3 Rest Period: 30 to 45 seconds between exercises				No. of sets: 2
	Russian Twist (feet crossed and elevated)	98	15	12
Cool Down/Stretch				

SILVER PROGRAM, Week 3, Saturday				
	Exercise	**Page #**	**Weight**	**No. of Reps**
Warm-up				
Drill 1 Rest Period: up to 1 minute after 2 exercises are completed				No. of sets: 1
	Double Arm Swing	58	20	20
	Swing Clean	81	20	10 each
Drill 2 Rest Period: up to 45 seconds after 2 exercises are completed				No. of sets: 1
	Double Arm Swing	58	20	15

SILVER PROGRAM, Week 3, Saturday				
	Exercise	**Page #**	**Weight**	**No. of Reps**
	Swing Clean	81	20	8 each

Drill 3
Rest Period: up to 30 seconds after 2 exercises are completed   No. of sets: 1

	Double Arm Swing	58	20	10
	Swing Clean	81	20	5 each

Drill 4
Rest Period: n/a   No. of sets: 1

	Double Arm Swing	58	20	10
	Swing Clean	81	20	5 each

Cool Down/Stretch

SILVER PROGRAM, Week 4, Monday				
	Exercise	**Page #**	**Weight**	**No. of Reps**
Warm-up				

Drill 1
Rest Period: 45 seconds to 1 minute after 2 exercises are completed   No. of sets: 2

	Exercise	Page #	Weight	No. of Reps
	Rack Squat	48	15	12 each
	Overhead Press, Elbow to Knee	79	15	10 each

Drill 2
Rest Period: 45 seconds to 1 minute after 2 exercises are complete   No. of sets: 2

	Exercise	Page #	Weight	No. of Reps
	Swing Clean	81	15	10 each
	Swing to Right Angle, Bottom Up	80	15	10 each

Drill 3
Rest Period: 45 seconds to 1 minute after 2 exercises are completed   No. of sets: 2

	Exercise	Page #	Weight	No. of Reps
	Windmill—No Kettlebell	86	n/a	10 each

SILVER PROGRAM, Week 4, Monday				
	Exercise	Page #	Weight	No. of Reps
	Single Arm Swing	60	15	15 each
Drill 4 Rest Period: 45 seconds to 1 minute after 2 exercises are completed No. of sets: 2				
	Overhead/Chest/Situp/Press	99	15	12 each
Cool Down/Stretch				

SILVER PROGRAM, Week 4, Wednesday				
	Exercise	Page #	Weight	No. of Reps
Warm-up				
Drill 1 Rest Period: 30 to 45 seconds between exercises No. of sets: 2				
	Halo	51	15	10 each
	Double Arm Swing	58	15	20

SILVER PROGRAM, Week 4, Wednesday				
	Exercise	**Page #**	**Weight**	**No. of Reps**
Drill 2 Rest Period: 30 to 45 seconds between exercises			No. of sets: 2	
	Lateral Lunge, Open Arm	54	15	12 each
	Bent Over Row	70	15	15 each
Drill 3 Rest Period: 30 to 45 seconds between exercises			No. of sets: 1	
	Turkish Get Up Prep	95	15	6 each
	Russian Twist (feet crossed and elevated)	98	15	15
Cool Down/Stretch				

Body Sculpting *with* **Kettlebells**

	Exercise	Page #	Weight	No. of Reps
SILVER PROGRAM, Week 4, Friday				
Warm-up				
Drill 1				
Rest Period: 45 seconds to 1 minute between exercises				No. of sets: 2
	Rack Squat	48	20	8 each
	Backward Lunge with Pass	53	20	8 each
Drill 2				
Rest Period: 45 seconds to 1 minute between exercises				No. of sets: 2
	Swing Clean	81	20	6 each
	Stay in Squat Figure 8	78	20	8
Drill 3				
Rest Period: 45 seconds to 1 minute between exercises				No. of sets: 2
	Romanian Dead Lift	73	20	12

SILVER PROGRAM, Week 4, Friday				
	Exercise	**Page #**	**Weight**	**No. of Reps**
	Push-up (straight legs)	76	n/a	8, 6

Drill 4				
Rest Period: 45 seconds to 1 minute between exercises			No. of sets: 1	
	Plank Row, Pass	100	15	8 each

Cool Down/Stretch

SILVER PROGRAM, Week 4, Saturday				
	Exercise	**Page #**	**Weight**	**No. of Reps**
Warm-up				

Drill 1				
Rest Period: up to 90 seconds after 3 exercises are completed			No. of sets: 3	
	Overhead Press, Elbow to Knee	79	15	10 each
	Lateral Lunge, Open Arm	54	15	10 each
	Single Arm Swing	60	15	15 each

Cool Down/Stretch

SILVER PROGRAM, Week 5, Monday				
	Exercise	**Page #**	**Weight**	**No. of Reps**
Warm-up				
Drill 1				
Rest Period: 45 seconds to 1 minute between exercises				No. of sets: 3
	Rack Squat, Swing Clean	48, 81	20	8 each
	Double Arm High Pull	66	20	15
	Double Arm Swing	58	20	15
Drill 2				
Rest Period: 45 seconds to 1 minute between exercises				No. of sets: 3
	Backward Lunge with Pass (alternating)	53	20	10 each
	Bent Over Row	70	20	15 each

SILVER PROGRAM, Week 5, Monday				
	Exercise	**Page #**	**Weight**	**No. of Reps**
	Tricep Press with Balance	71	20	8 each leg

Drill 3
Rest Period: 45 seconds to 1 minute between exercises   No. of sets: 2

	Russian Twist (feet on floor, knees bent)	98	20	15
	Overhead/Chest/Sit Up/ Press	99	15	15

Cool Down/Stretch

SILVER PROGRAM, Week 5, Wednesday				
	Exercise	**Page #**	**Weight**	**No. of Reps**

Warm-up

Drill 1
Rest Period: 30 seconds between exercises   No. of sets: 3

	Rack Squat	48	15	15 each
	Overhead Press, Elbow to Knee	79	15	12 each

Body Sculpting *with* **Kettlebells**

SILVER PROGRAM, Week 5, Wednesday

	Exercise	Page #	Weight	No. of Reps
	Lateral Lunge, Open Arm	54	15	10 each
	Swing Clean	81	15	15 each

Drill 2
Rest Period: 30 seconds between exercises   No. of sets: 2

	Exercise	Page #	Weight	No. of Reps
	Overhead/Chest/Situp/Press	99	15	15
	Turkish Get Up Prep	95	15	8 each

Cool Down/Stretch

SILVER PROGRAM, Week 5, Friday

	Exercise	Page #	Weight	No. of Reps
Warm-up				

Drill 1
Rest Period: 30 to 45 seconds between exercises   No. of sets: 3

	Exercise	Page #	Weight	No. of Reps
	Halo	51	15	10 each

SILVER PROGRAM, Week 5, Friday				
	Exercise	**Page #**	**Weight**	**No. of Reps**
	Double Arm Swing	58	15	15
	Swing to Right Angle, Bottom Up	80	15	10 each

Drill 2
Rest Period: 30 to 45 seconds between exercises   No. of sets: 3

	Exercise	Page #	Weight	No. of Reps
	Windmill with Bicep Curl	88	15	8 each
	Push-up (straight legs)	76	15	6, 4, 3
	Vertical Clean	83	15	15 each

Drill 3
Rest Period: 30 to 45 seconds between exercises   No. of sets: 2

	Exercise	Page #	Weight	No. of Reps
	Russian Twist (feet crossed and elevated)	98	15	15

Cool Down/Stretch

SILVER PROGRAM, Week 5, Saturday

	Exercise	Page #	Weight	No. of Reps
Warm-up				
Drill 1				
Rest Period: up to 45 seconds after 2 exercises are completed			No. of sets: 4	
	Rack Squat, Swing Clean	48, 81	20	10 each
	Double Arm Swing	58	20	20
Cool Down/Stretch				

SILVER PROGRAM, Week 6, Monday

	Exercise	Page #	Weight	No. of Reps
Warm-up				
Drill 1				
Rest Period: 30 seconds between exercises			No. of sets: 3	
	Rack Squat, Press	50	15	15 each
	Swing Clean	81	15	10 each
	Single Arm Swing with Hand Switch	62	15	10 each

SILVER PROGRAM, Week 6, Monday				
	Exercise	**Page #**	**Weight**	**No. of Reps**
	Windmill with Bicep Curl (kettlebell at lower hand)	88	15	10 each

Drill 2
Rest Period: 30 seconds between exercises   No. of sets: 2

	Exercise	**Page #**	**Weight**	**No. of Reps**
	Overhead/ Chest/ Situp/ Press	99	15	15
	Turkish Get Up Prep	95	15	8 each

Cool Down/Stretch

SILVER PROGRAM, Week 6, Wednesday				
	Exercise	**Page #**	**Weight**	**No. of Reps**

Warm-up

Drill 1
Rest Period: up to 1 minute after 2 exercises are completed   No. of sets: 3

	Exercise	**Page #**	**Weight**	**No. of Reps**
	Rack Squat	48	20	8 each
	Backward Lunge with Pass	53	20	8 each

	Exercise	Page #	Weight	No. of Reps
SILVER PROGRAM, Week 6, Wednesday				
Drill 2 Rest Period: up to 1 minute after 2 exercises are completed				No. of sets: 3
	Swing Clean	81	20	8 each
	Stay in Squat Figure 8	78	20	8 each
Drill 3 Rest Period: up to 1 minute after 2 exercises are completed				No. of sets: 3
	Romanian Dead Lift	73	20	12
	Push-up (straight legs)	76	n/a	6, 5, 4
Drill 4 Rest Period: up to 1 minute after 2 exercises are completed				No. of sets: 2
	Russian Twist (feet crossed and elevated)	98	20	10

SILVER PROGRAM, Week 6, Wednesday				
	Exercise	**Page #**	**Weight**	**No. of Reps**
	Plank Row, Pass	100	15	10, 8
Cool Down/Stretch				

SILVER PROGRAM, Week 6, Friday				
	Exercise	**Page #**	**Weight**	**No. of Reps**
Warm-up				
Drill 1 Rest Period: 30 to 45 seconds between exercises				No. of sets: 3
	Halo	51	15	10 each
	Single Arm Swing	60	15	15 each
Drill 2 Rest Period: 30 to 45 seconds between exercises				No. of sets: 3
	Lateral Lunge, Open Arm, Press	55	15	12 each
	Bent Over Row	70	15	15 each

SILVER PROGRAM, Week 6, Friday				
	Exercise	**Page #**	**Weight**	**No. of Reps**
Drill 3 Rest Period: 30 to 45 seconds between exercises				No. of sets: 2
	Russian Twist (feet crossed and elevated)	98	15	15
	Turkish Get Up Prep	95	15	8 each
	Clam	102	15	15
Cool Down/Stretch				

SILVER PROGRAM, Week 6, Saturday				
	Exercise	**Page #**	**Weight**	**No. of Reps**
Warm-up				
Drill 1 Rest Period: up to 45 seconds after 2 exercises are completed				No. of sets: 3
	Forward Walking Lunge with Pass	53	20	15
	Tricep Press with Balance	71	20	10 (change legs after 5 reps)
Cool Down/Stretch				

Gold Medal Program

11

Program Level: 2
Program Length: 6 weeks, 4 workouts per week.
Weight: 15 lb, 20 lb, and 25 lb kettlebells
Workout Length: Approximately 45-60 minutes.

This level introduces combinations of existing exercises. The fourth day of each week is a super-set day of shorter duration than days 1-3 and introduces timed drills for endurance, cardio, and fat loss.

GOLD PROGRAM, Week 1, Monday				
	Exercise	**Page #**	**Weight**	**No. of Reps**
Warm-up				
Drill 1				
Rest Period: 45 seconds to 1 minute between exercises				No. of sets: 3
	Rack Squat	48	20	10 each
	Push Press	82	20	6 each
	Double Arm Swing	58	20	15
Drill 2				
Rest Period: 45 seconds to 1 minute between exercises				No. of sets: 3
	Backward Lunge with Pass	53	20	8 each
	Bent Over Row	70	20	12 each
	Push-up (on knees, if necessary)	76	n/a	10, 8, 6

GOLD PROGRAM, Week 1, Monday				
	Exercise	**Page #**	**Weight**	**No. of Reps**
Drill 3				
Rest Period: up to 45 seconds between exercises				No. of sets: 2
	Russian Twist (feet crossed and elevated)	98	20	10
Cool Down/Stretch				

GOLD PROGRAM, Week 1, Wednesday				
Warm-up				
Drill 1				
Rest Period: 45 seconds to 1 minute after 2 exercises are completed				No. of sets: 3
	Hanging Straight Arm Squat, Vertical Clean (1 Squat + 1 Vertical Clean = 1 rep)	47, 83	20	8 each
	Squat/Stand Figure 8 with Balance	78	20	8
Drill 2				
Rest Period: 45 seconds to 1 minute after 2 exercises are completed				No. of sets: 3
	Windmill with Lower Kettlebell Lift	87	20	8 each
	Double Arm Swing	58	20	15

GOLD PROGRAM, Week 1, Wednesday				
	Exercise	**Page #**	**Weight**	**No. of Reps**
Drill 3 Rest Period: 45 seconds to 1 minute after 2 exercises are completed				No. of sets: 2
	Russian Twist (feet crossed and elevated)	98	20	15
	Plank Row, Pass	100	20	8
Cool Down/Stretch				

GOLD PROGRAM, Week 1, Friday				
	Exercise	**Page #**	**Weight**	**No. of Reps**
Warm-up				
Drill 1 Rest Period: 30 to 45 seconds between exercises				No. of sets: 3
	Rack Squat, Press	50	15	15 each
	Single Arm High Pull with Switches	69	15	10 each
	Tricep Press with Alternating Backward Lunge	72	15	10 each

GOLD PROGRAM, Week 1, Friday

	Exercise	Page #	Weight	No. of Reps
	Single Arm Swing	60	15	15 each
	Forward Walking Lunge with Pass	53	15	15 each
	Turkish Get Up Prep	95	15	8 each
	Plank Row, Pass	100	15	10

Cool Down/Stretch

GOLD PROGRAM, Week 1, Saturday

	Exercise	Page #	Weight	Time
Warm-up				
Drill 1 Rest Period: up to 45 seconds between drills				
	Double Arm Swing	58	20	1 minute

GOLD PROGRAM, Week 1, Saturday				
	Exercise	**Page #**	**Weight**	**Time**
Drill 2				
Rest Period: up to 45 seconds between drills				No. of sets: 3
	Swing Clean	81	20	30 seconds each (no less than 10 reps every 30 seconds)
Cool Down/Stretch				

GOLD PROGRAM, Week 2, Monday				
	Exercise	**Page #**	**Weight**	**No. of Reps**
Warm-up				
Drill 1				
Rest Period: up to 1 minute after 2 exercises are completed				No. of sets: 2
	Rack Squat	48	25	6 each
Swing Clean to Push Press		81, 82	25	5 each
Drill 2				
Rest Period: up to 1 minute after 2 exercises are completed				No. of sets: 2
	Romanian Dead Lift	73	25	8

GOLD PROGRAM, Week 2, Monday				
	Exercise	**Page #**	**Weight**	**No. of Reps**
	Double Arm Swing	58	25	8

Drill 3

Rest Period: up to 1 minute after 2 exercises are completed   No. of sets: 2

	Backward Lunge with Pass	53	25	6 each
	Torso Circles	94	25	8 each

Drill 4

Rest Period: n/a   No. of sets: 1

	Russian Twist (feet crossed and elevated)	98	15	15

Cool Down/Stretch

GOLD PROGRAM, Week 2, Wednesday				
	Exercise	**Page #**	**Weight**	**No. of Reps**
Drill 1				
Rest Period: 45 seconds to 1 minute between exercises				No. of sets: 3
	Hanging Straight Arm Squat, Vertical Clean(1 Squat + 1 Vertical Clean = 1 rep)	47, 83	20	10, 8, 6
	Single Arm Swing	60	20	15 each
Drill 2				
Rest Period: 45 seconds to 1 minute between exercises				No. of sets: 3
	Windmill with Lower Kettlebell Lift (no kettlebell overhead)	87	20	8 each
	Forward Walking Lunge with Pass	53	20	15 each
Drill 3				
Rest Period: 45 seconds to 1 minute between exercises				No. of sets: 2
	Russian Twist (feet crossed and elevated)	98	20	15

GOLD PROGRAM, Week 2, Wednesday				
	Exercise	**Page #**	**Weight**	**No. of Reps**
	Plank Row, Pass	100	20	8
	Turkish Get Up Prep	95	20	8 each
Cool Down/Stretch				

GOLD PROGRAM, Week 2, Friday				
	Exercise	**Page #**	**Weight**	**No. of Reps**
Warm-up				
Drill 1 Rest Period: up to 1 minute after 2 exercises are completed				No. of sets: 3
	Single Arm Swing	60	15	15 each
	Swing Snatch	63	15	15 each
Drill 2 Rest Period: up to 1 minute after 2 exercises are completed				No. of sets: 3
	Single Arm High Pull with Switches	69	15	10 each

Body Sculpting *with* **Kettlebells**

GOLD PROGRAM, Week 2, Friday				
	Exercise	**Page #**	**Weight**	**No. of Reps**
	Push-up	76	n/a	12, 10, 8
Drill 3				
Rest Period: up to 1 minute after 2 exercises are completed				No. of sets: 3
	Full Turkish Get Up	96	15	2 each direction
	Plank Row, Pass	100	15	10
Cool Down/Stretch				

GOLD PROGRAM, Week 2, Saturday				
	Exercise	**Page #**	**Weight**	**Time**
Warm-up				
Drill 1				
Rest Period: up to 90 seconds after completing each side				No. of sets: n/a
Vertical Clean to Push Press		85	20	1 minute (no less than 12 reps per minute)

GOLD PROGRAM, Week 2, Saturday				
	Exercise	**Page #**	**Weight**	**Time**
Drill 2 Rest Period: up to 45 seconds				No. of sets: 3
	Side Plank Row, Pass	101	20	1 minute (no less than 10 reps per minute)
Cool Down/Stretch				

GOLD PROGRAM, Week 3, Monday				
	Exercise	**Page #**	**Weight**	**No. of Reps**
Warm-up				
Drill 1 Rest Period: 30 seconds between exercises				No. of sets: 3
	Double Arm Swing to Single Arm Swing	58, 60	15	double: 15, single: 10
	Overhead Press, Elbow to Knee	79	15	15 each
	Swing Snatch	63	15	15 each
	Windmill with Overhead Kettlebell	89	15	8 each

GOLD PROGRAM, Week 3, Monday				
	Exercise	**Page #**	**Weight**	**No. of Reps**
	Plank Row, Pass	100	15	10
Drill 2 Rest Period: up to 90 seconds between exercises				No. of sets: 2
	Full Turkish Get Up	96	15	3 each
Cool Down/Stretch				

GOLD PROGRAM, Week 3, Wednesday				
	Exercise	**Page #**	**Weight**	**No. of Reps**
Warm-up				
Drill 1 Rest Period: 45 seconds to 1 minute after 2 exercises are completed				No. of sets: 3
	Hanging Straight Arm Squat, Vertical Clean	47, 83	20	12, 10, 8
	Single Arm Swing	60	20	15 each
Drill 2 Rest Period: 45 seconds to 1 minute after 2 exercises are completed				No. of sets: 3
	One Legged Dead Lift, Touch Handle	75	20	10 each

GOLD PROGRAM, Week 3, Wednesday

	Exercise	Page #	Weight	No. of Reps
	Forward Walking Lunge with Pass	53	20	15 each

Drill 3
Rest Period: 45 seconds to 1 minute after 2 exercises are completed   No. of sets: 2

	Exercise	Page #	Weight	No. of Reps
	Overhead/Chest/Situp/Press	99	20	15
	Russian Twist (feet crossed and elevated)	98	20	15

Cool Down/Stretch

GOLD PROGRAM, Week 3, Friday

	Exercise	Page #	Weight	No. of Reps

Warm-up

Drill 1
Rest Period: up to 45 seconds between exercises   No. of sets: 3

	Exercise	Page #	Weight	No. of Reps
	Rack Squat	48	25	8 each
	Backward Lunge with Pass	53	25	6 each

GOLD PROGRAM, Week 3, Friday				
	Exercise	Page #	Weight	No. of Reps
Drill 2 Rest Period: up to 45 seconds between exercises			No. of sets: 3	
	Romanian Dead Lift	73	25	10
	Torso Circles	94	25	10 each
Drill 3 Rest Period: up to 45 seconds between exercises			No. of sets: 3	
	Double Arm High Pull	66	25	10
	Double Arm Swing	58	25	15
Drill 4 Rest Period: up to 45 seconds between exercises			No. of sets: 2	
	Clam	102	15	15

GOLD PROGRAM, Week 3, Friday				
	Exercise	**Page #**	**Weight**	**No. of Reps**
	Turkish Get Up Prep	95	15	10 each
Cool Down/Stretch				

GOLD PROGRAM, Week 3, Saturday				
	Exercise	**Page #**	**Weight**	**Time**
Warm-up				
Drill 1 Rest Period: up to 30 seconds between exercises			No. of sets: n/a	
	Single Arm Swing, Swing Clean	60, 81	20	1 minute each
Drill 2 Rest Period: up to 30 seconds between exercises			No. of sets: 3	
	Russian Twist (feet crossed and elevated)	98	20	30 seconds
Cool Down/Stretch				

GOLD PROGRAM, Week 4, Monday				
	Exercise	**Page #**	**Weight**	**No. of Reps**
Warm-up				
Drill 1				
Rest Period: 45 seconds to 1 minute between exercises			No. of sets: 3	
	Hanging Straight Arm Squat, Vertical Clean (1 Squat + 1 Vertical Clean = 1 rep)	47, 83	20	15, 12, 8
	Single Arm Swing	60	20	15 each
Drill 2				
Rest Period: 45 seconds to 1 minute between exercises			No. of sets: 3	
	Windmill with Overhead Kettlebell	89	20	10, 8, 5
	Forward Walking Lunge with Pass	53	20	15 each
Drill 3				
Rest Period: 45 seconds to 1 minute between exercises			No. of sets: 3	
	Single Arm High Pull (one side at a time, no switch)	69	20	10, 8, 5

GOLD PROGRAM, Week 4, Monday

	Exercise	Page #	Weight	No. of Reps
	One Legged Dead Lift with Kettlebell	75	20	10 each

Drill 4
Rest Period: 45 seconds to 1 minute between exercises   No. of sets: 2

	Exercise	Page #	Weight	No. of Reps
	Russian Twist (feet crossed and elevated)	98	20	15

Cool Down/Stretch

GOLD PROGRAM, Week 4, Wednesday

	Exercise	Page #	Weight	No. of Reps
Warm-up				

Drill 1
Rest Period: 30 seconds between exercises   No. of sets: 3

	Exercise	Page #	Weight	No. of Reps
Swing Clean, Press, Overhead Squat		81, 49, 91	15	12, 8, 6
	Swing to Right Angle, Bottom Up	80	15	15 each
	Single Arm Swing with Hand Switch	62	15	15 each

	Exercise	Page #	Weight	No. of Reps
GOLD PROGRAM, Week 4, Wednesday				
	Side Plank Row, Pass	101	15	8
	Overhead/Chest/Situp/Press	99	15	15
Cool Down/Stretch				

	Exercise	Page #	Weight	No. of Reps
GOLD PROGRAM, Week 4, Friday				
Warm-up				
Drill 1 Rest Period: 45 seconds to 1 minute after 2 exercises are completed				No. of sets: 3
	Double Arm Swing to Single Arm Swing	58, 60	15	double: 15, single: 10
	Lateral Lunge, Open Arm with Press	55	15	12, 8, 6
Drill 2 Rest Period: 45 seconds to 1 minute after 2 exercises are completed				No. of sets: 3
	Halo	51	15	10 each

GOLD PROGRAM, Week 4, Friday

	Exercise	Page #	Weight	No. of Reps
	Single Arm High Pull with Switches	69	15	10 each

Drill 3
Rest Period: up to 90 seconds after both sides are completed · · · · · · No. of sets: 3

	Exercise	Page #	Weight	No. of Reps
		96, 63	15	3 each
3 Full Turkish Get Ups with 5 Swing Snatches (TGU, once standing perform 5 Swing Snatches, then return to floor)				

Cool Down/Stretch

GOLD PROGRAM, Week 4, Saturday

	Exercise	Page #	Weight	Time
Warm-up				

Drill 1
Rest Period: up to 45 seconds after 2 exercises are completed · · · · · · No. of sets: 5

	Exercise	Page #	Weight	Time
	Double Arm Swing	58	25	30 seconds
	Push-up (on knees if neccessary)	76	n/a	30 seconds (no less than 10 reps in 30 seconds)

Cool Down/Stretch

GOLD PROGRAM, Week 5, Monday				
	Exercise	**Page #**	**Weight**	**No. of Reps**
Warm-up				
Drill 1				
Rest Period: 30 seconds between exercises			No. of sets: 3	
	Overhead Press, Elbow to Knee	79	15	15 each
	Single Arm Swing	60	15	15 each
	Bent Over Row	70	15	20 each
	Two Kettlebell Windmill (15 lb overhead, 20 lb below, lift 20 lb upon standing upright)	90	15 & 20	8 each side
	Russian Twist (feet crossed and elevated)	98	15	15
Cool Down/Stretch				

GOLD PROGRAM, Week 5, Wednesday				
	Exercise	**Page #**	**Weight**	**No. of Reps**
Warm-up				
Drill 1				
Rest Period: 45 seconds to 1 minute after 2 exercises are completed			No. of sets: 3	
	Straight Arm Squat to Vertical Clean	47, 83	20	12, 10, 8
	Single Arm Swing	60	20	15 each
Drill 2				
Rest Period: 45 seconds to 1 minute after 2 exercises are completed			No. of sets: 3	
	One Legged Dead Lift with Kettlebell	75	20	10 each
	Forward Walking Lunge with Pass	53	20	15 each
Drill 3				
Rest Period: 45 seconds to 1 minute after 2 exercises are completed			No. of sets: 3	
	Overhead/Chest/Situp/Press	99	20	10

GOLD PROGRAM, Week 5, Wednesday				
	Exercise	**Page #**	**Weight**	**No. of Reps**
	Plank Row, Pass	100	20	10
Cool Down/Stretch				

GOLD PROGRAM, Week 5, Friday				
	Exercise	**Page #**	**Weight**	**No. of Reps**
Warm-up				
Drill 1				
Rest Period: up to 45 seconds between exercises			No. of sets: 3	
	Rack Squat	48	25	8 each
	Backward Lunge with Pass	53	25	6 each
Drill 2				
Rest Period: up to 45 seconds between exercises			No. of sets: 3	
	Romanian Dead Lift	73	25	10
	Torso Circles	94	25	10 each

GOLD PROGRAM, Week 5, Friday

	Exercise	Page #	Weight	No. of Reps
Drill 3 Rest Period: up to 45 seconds between exercises			No. of sets: 3	
	Double Arm High Pull	66	25	10
	Double Arm Swing	58	25	15
Drill 4 Rest Period: up to 45 seconds between exercises			No. of sets: 2	
	Clam	102	15	15
	Full Turkish Get Up (up to 2 minutes)	96	15	5 each
Cool Down/Stretch				

GOLD PROGRAM, Week 5, Saturday

	Exercise	Page #	Weight	Time
Warm-up				
Drill 1 Rest Period: up to 1 minute after completing both sides			No. of sets: 3	
	Swing Clean to Push Press to Overhead Squat	81, 82, 91	20	1 minute each side (no less than 10 reps per minute)

GOLD PROGRAM, Week 5, Saturday

	Exercise	Page #	Weight	Time
Drill 2 Rest Period: up to 1 minute after 2 exercises are completed				No. of sets: 3
	Side Plank Row, Pass	101	20	1 minute (no less than 10 reps per minute)
Cool Down/Stretch				

GOLD PROGRAM, Week 6, Monday

	Exercise	Page #	Weight	No. of Reps
Warm-up				
Drill 1 Rest Period: 45 seconds to 1 minute after 2 exercises are completed				No. of sets: 2
	Rack Squat	48	25	6 each
Swing Clean, Push Press		81, 82	25	6 each
Drill 2 Rest Period: 45 seconds to 1 minute after 2 exercises are completed				No. of sets: 2
	Romanian Dead Lift	73	25	10

GOLD PROGRAM, Week 6, Monday

	Exercise	Page #	Weight	No. of Reps
	Double Arm Swing	58	25	10

Drill 3
Rest Period: 45 seconds to 1 minute after 2 exercises are completed   No. of sets: 2

	Exercise	Page #	Weight	No. of Reps
	Backward Lunge with Pass	53	25	6 each
	Torso Circles	94	25	10 each

Drill 4
Rest Period: 45 seconds to 1 minute after 2 exercises are completed   No. of sets: 2

	Exercise	Page #	Weight	No. of Reps
	Russian Twist (feet crossed and elevated)	98	15	15
	Overhead/Chest/Situp/Press	99	15	15

Cool Down/Stretch

GOLD PROGRAM, Week 6, Wednesday				
	Exercise	**Page #**	**Weight**	**No. of Reps**
Warm-up				
Drill 1				
Rest Period: 45 seconds to 1 minute between exercises			No. of sets: 2	
	Two Kettlebells: One Press, One Push Press (1 Press + 1 Push Press = 1 rep)	84	15 (Press) & 20 (Push Press)	5 each side
	Swing to Right Angle, Bottom Up	80	20	10 each
Drill 2				
Rest Period: 45 seconds to 1 minute between exercises			No. of sets: 2	
	Windmill with Lower Kettlebell Lift	87	20	15 each
	Forward Walking Lunge with Pass	53	20	15 each
Drill 3				
Rest Period: 45 seconds to 1 minute between exercises			No. of sets: 2	
	Plank Row, Pass	100	20	8

GOLD PROGRAM, Week 6, Wednesday

	Exercise	Page #	Weight	No. of Reps
	Clam	102	15	15

Cool Down/Stretch

GOLD PROGRAM, Week 6, Friday

	Exercise	Page #	Weight	No. of Reps
Warm-up				

Drill 1
Rest Period: 45 seconds to 1 minute after 2 exercises are completed   No. of sets: 2

	Exercise	Page #	Weight	No. of Reps
	Single Arm Swing	60	15	10 each
	Single Arm High Pull with Switches	69	15	10 each

Drill 2
Rest Period: 45 seconds to 1 minute after 2 exercises are completed   No. of sets: 2

	Exercise	Page #	Weight	No. of Reps
	Halo	51	15	10 each
	Lateral Lunge, Open Arm with Press	55	15	10 each

GOLD PROGRAM, Week 6, Friday				
	Exercise	**Page #**	**Weight**	**No. of Reps**
Drill 3 Rest Period: 45 seconds to 1 minute after 2 exercises are completed No. of sets: 2				
	Squat/Stand Figure 8 with Balance	78	15	15 each
	Swing Snatch	63	15	15 each
Drill 4 Rest Period: 45 seconds to 1 minute after 2 exercises are completed No. of sets: 2				
	Full Turkish Get Up	96	15	3 each
	Russian Twist (feet crossed and elevated)	98	15	20
Cool Down/Stretch				

GOLD PROGRAM, Week 6, Saturday				
	Exercise	**Page #**	**Weight**	**Time**
Warm-up				
Drill 1				
Rest Period: up to 45 seconds after 2 exercises are completed			No. of sets: 3	
	Double Arm Swing	58	25	1 minute
Drill 2				
Rest Period: up to 45 seconds after 2 exercises are completed			No. of sets: 3	
	Double Arm High Pull	66	25	30 seconds
Drill 3				
Rest Period: up to 45 seconds after 2 exercises are completed			No. of sets: 3	
	Push-up (on knees if neccessary)	76	n/a	30 seconds (no less than 10 reps in 30 seconds)
Cool Down/Stretch				

Platinum Medal Program

12

Program Level: 3
Program Length: 6 weeks, 4 workouts per week.
Weight: 15 lb, 20 lb, and 25 lb kettlebells
Workout Length: Approximately 45-60 minutes.

This Program includes more super-sets to increase strength, cardio and endurance. Timed drills continue on the fourth day of each week, and these workouts will be of shorter duration than days 1 – 3.

REMEMBER: Always maintain proper skills! If your form begins to break down, stop for the day, or take a few minutes to rest and then resume the workout with a lighter bell.

PLATINUM PROGRAM, Week 1, Monday				
	Exercise	**Page #**	**Weight**	**No. of Reps**
Warm-up				
Drill 1				
Rest Period: 45 seconds to 1 minute after 2 exercises are completed				No. of sets: 3
	Vertical Clean, Rack Squat	83, 48	25	8 each
	Double Arm High Pull	66	25	10
Drill 2				
Rest Period: 45 seconds to 1 minute after 2 exercises are completed				No. of sets: 3
	Romanian Dead Lift	73	25	10
	Single Arm Swing (low; navel height)	60	25	10 each
Drill 3				
Rest Period: 45 seconds to 1 minute after 2 exercises are completed				No. of sets: 3
	Stay in Squat Figure 8	78	25	10

PLATINUM PROGRAM, Week 1, Monday				
	Exercise	**Page #**	**Weight**	**No. of Reps**
	Torso Circles	94	25	12 each
Drill 4				
Rest Period: 45 seconds to 1 minute after 2 exercises are completed			No. of sets: 3	
	Russian Twist (slow; knees bent and feet on floor)	98	25	8
Russian Twist (feet crossed and elevated)		98	15	20
Cool Down/Stretch				

PLATINUM PROGRAM, Week 1, Wednesday				
	Exercise	**Page #**	**Weight**	**No. of Reps**
Warm-up				
Drill 1				
Rest Period: 45 seconds to 1 minute between exercises			No. of sets: 3	
Two Kettlebells: One Press, One Push Press (1 Press + 1 Push Press = 1 rep)		84	15 (Press), 20 (Push Press)	8 each
	Swing Clean	82	20	15 each

PLATINUM PROGRAM, Week 1, Wednesday				
	Exercise	**Page #**	**Weight**	**No. of Reps**
Drill 2				
Rest Period: 45 seconds to 1 minute between exercises				No. of sets: 3
	Forward Walking Lunge with Pass	53	20	15 each
	Double Arm Swing, Step-Step	64	20	15
Drill 3				
Rest Period: 45 seconds to 1 minute between exercises				No. of sets: 3
	Plank Row, Pass	100	20	8
	Russian Twist (feet crossed and elevated)	98	20	15
Cool Down/Stretch				

PLATINUM PROGRAM, Week 1, Friday				
	Exercise	**Page #**	**Weight**	**No. of Reps**
Warm-up				
Drill 1 Rest Period: up to 90 seconds				No. of sets: 3
	Vertical Clean, Press, Windmill with Overhead Kettlebell (after Windmill, return bell to rack position, then lower straight arm to prepare for next vertical clean)	83, 49, 89	15	15, 12, 8
	Bent Over Row	70	15	20 each
	One Legged Dead Lift with Kettlebell	75	15	15 each
	Side Plank Row, Pass	101	15	10
	Full Turkish Get Up	96	15	3 each

PLATINUM PROGRAM, Week 1, Friday				
	Exercise	**Page #**	**Weight**	**No. of Reps**
Drill 2 Rest Period: 30 seconds between exercises				No. of sets: 3
	Clam	102	15	15
Cool Down/Stretch				

PLATINUM PROGRAM, Week 1, Saturday				
	Exercise	**Page #**	**Weight**	**Time**
Warm-up				
Drill 1 Rest Period: up to 2 minutes , No. of sets: 3				
	Swing Clean	82	20	3 minutes (alternate arms every 30 seconds)
Drill 2 Rest Period: up to 60 seconds				No. of sets: 3
	Swing Snatch	63	20	2 minutes (alternate arms every 30 seconds)
Drill 3 Rest Period: up to 60 seconds				No. of sets: 3
	Russian Twist (feet crossed and elevated)	98	20	30 seconds
Cool Down/Stretch				

PLATINUM PROGRAM, Week 2, Monday				
	Exercise	**Page #**	**Weight**	**No. of Reps**
Warm-up				
Drill 1 Rest Period: 30 to 45 seconds between exercises				No. of sets: 3
	Two Kettlebells: One Press, One Push Press (1 Press + 1 Push Press = 1 rep)	84	15, 20	8 each
	Single Arm Swing, Swing Clean	60, 82	20	10 each
Drill 2 Rest Period: 30 to 45 seconds between exercises				No. of sets: 3
	Forward Walking Lunge with Pass	53	20	15 each
	Double Arm Swing, Step-Step	64	20	15
Drill 3 Rest Period: 30 to 45 seconds between exercises				No. of sets: 2
	Plank Row, Pass	100	20	10

PLATINUM PROGRAM, Week 2, Monday				
	Exercise	**Page #**	**Weight**	**No. of Reps**
	Russian Twist (feet crossed and elevated)	98	20	15
	Overhead/Chest/Situp/Press	99	15	15
Cool Down/Stretch				

PLATINUM PROGRAM, Week 2, Wednesday				
	Exercise	**Page #**	**Weight**	**No. of Reps**
Warm-up				
Drill 1				
Rest Period: 1 minute to 90 seconds after 2 exercises are completed				No. of sets: 3
	Vertical Clean, Rack Squat	83, 48	25	10, 8, 6
	Double Arm Swing	58	25	12

PLATINUM PROGRAM, Week 2, Wednesday				
	Exercise	**Page #**	**Weight**	**No. of Reps**
Drill 2 Rest Period: 1 minute to 90 seconds after 2 exercises are completed No. of sets: 3				
	Romanian Dead Lift	73	25	12
	Swing Snatch	63	20	12 each
Drill 3 Rest Period: 1 minute to 90 seconds after 2 exercises are completed No. of sets: 3				
	Stay in Squat Figure 8	78	25	10, 8, 6
	Torso Circles	94	25	12 each
Drill 4 Rest Period: 45 seconds between exercises No. of sets: 2				
	Russian Twist (feet crossed and elevated)	98	20	8
Cool Down/Stretch				

PLATINUM PROGRAM, Week 2, Friday				
	Exercise	Page #	Weight	No. of Reps
Warm-up				
Drill 1 Rest Period: 45 seconds to 1 minute between exercises				No. of sets: 3
	Double Arm Swing, Single Arm Swing, Swing with Switch	58, 60, 62	20	15 (Double), 10 (Single), 5 each (Switch)
	Swing Clean, Push Press, Windmill with Overhead Kettlebell*	85, 89	20	8, 6, 4
	Backward Lunge with Pass	53	20	15 each
	Vertical Clean, Single Arm High Pull (1 Clean + 1 Pull = 1 rep)	83, 69	20	10 each
Drill 2 Rest Period: 45 seconds to 1 minute between exercises				No. of sets: 1
	Full Turkish Get Up	96	20	4 each

PLATINUM PROGRAM, Week 2, Friday				
	Exercise	**Page #**	**Weight**	**No. of Reps**
	Plank Row, Pass	100	20	10
Cool Down/Stretch				

PLATINUM PROGRAM, Week 2, Saturday				
	Exercise	**Page #**	**Weight**	**Time**
Warm-up				
Drill 1 Rest Period: up to 2 minutes after completing both sides			No. of sets: 3	
	Swing Clean, Swing Snatch, Overhead Squat*	82, 63, 91	20	2 minutes each (no less than 12 reps each minute)
Drill 2 Rest Period: up to 30 seconds between drills			No. of sets: 3	
	Single Arm High Pull with Switches	69	20	30 seconds
Cool Down/Stretch				

* Images should be read clock-wise.

PLATINUM PROGRAM, Week 3, Monday				
	Exercise	**Page #**	**Weight**	**No. of Reps**
Warm-up				
Drill 1				
Rest Period: up to 30 seconds after 2 exercises are completed			No. of sets: 3	
Vertical Clean with Push Press		85	25	8 each
	Double Arm Swing	58	25	12
Drill 2				
Rest Period: up to 30 seconds after 2 exercises are completed			No. of sets: 3	
	Romanian Dead Lift	73	25	12
	Single Arm Swing	60	20	12 each
Drill 3				
Rest Period: up to 30 seconds after 2 exercises are completed			No. of sets: 3	
	Stay in Squat Figure 8	78	25	10 each

PLATINUM PROGRAM, Week 3, Monday				
	Exercise	**Page #**	**Weight**	**No. of Reps**
	Torso Circles	94	25	12 each
Drill 4 Rest Period: up to 30 seconds, No. of sets: 2				
	Plank Row, Pass	100	20	10
Cool Down/Stretch				

PLATINUM PROGRAM, Week 3, Wednesday				
	Exercise	**Page #**	**Weight**	**No. of Reps**
Warm-up				
Drill 1 Rest Period: 30 to 45 seconds between exercises			No. of sets: 3	
	Single Arm Swing with Hand Switch	62	20	10 each
	Single Arm High Pull	69	20	10 each

PLATINUM PROGRAM, Week 3, Wednesday				
	Exercise	**Page #**	**Weight**	**No. of Reps**
Drill 2 Rest Period: 30 to 45 seconds between exercises				No. of sets: 3
	Forward Walking Lunge with Pass	53	20	15 each
	Swing Snatch to Windmill with Overhead Kettlebell	63, 89	20	10 each
Drill 3 Rest Period: 30 to 45 seconds between exercises				No. of sets: 3
	Full Turkish Get Up	92	15	3 each
	Overhead/Chest/Situp/Press	99	15	15
	Russian Twist (feet crossed and elevated)	98	20	15
Cool Down/Stretch				

PLATINUM PROGRAM, Week 3, Friday				
	Exercise	**Page #**	**Weight**	**No. of Reps**
Warm-up				
Drill 1				
Rest Period: 30 seconds between exercises				No. of sets: 3
	Rack Squat, Press	50	20	10, 8, 6
	Swing to Right Angle, Bottom Up	80	20	10 each
	Swing Clean, Push Press, Windmill with Overhead Kettlebell*	85, 89	20	8 each
	Side Plank Row, Pass	101	20	8 each
	Clam	102	15	15
Cool Down/Stretch				

* Images should be read clock-wise.

PLATINUM PROGRAM, Week 3, Saturday				
	Exercise	**Page #**	**Weight**	**Time**
Warm-up				
Drill 1 Rest Period: up to 90 seconds				No. of sets: 3
	Single Arm Swing	60	25	4 minutes (alternate arms every 30 seconds)
Drill 2 Rest Period: up to 45 seconds between drills				No. of sets: 3
	Backward Lunge with Pass	53	25	1 minute
Cool Down/Stretch				

PLATINUM PROGRAM, Week 4, Monday				
	Exercise	**Page #**	**Weight**	**Time**
Warm-up				
Drill 1 Rest Period: 30 to 45 seconds between exercises				No. of sets: 2
	Hanging Straight Arm Squat, Vertical Clean, Push Press*	47, 85	20	10, 8, 6
	Single Arm Swing, Swing Clean	60, 82		10 each

PLATINUM PROGRAM, Week 4, Monday				
	Exercise	**Page #**	**Weight**	**No. of Reps**
	Two Kettlebell Windmill	90	15 (overhead), 20 (below), 20 (upon standing upright)	10 each
	Bent Over Row	70	20	15 each
	Backward Lunge with Pass	53	20	10 each
	Swing Snatch	63	20	10 each
Drill 2				
Rest Period: 30 to 45 seconds between exercises			No. of sets: 1	
	Overhead/Chest/Situp/Press	99	15	20
Cool Down/Stretch				

* Images should be read clock-wise.

PLATINUM PROGRAM, Week 4, Wednesday				
	Exercise	**Page #**	**Weight**	**No. of Reps**
Warm-up				
Drill 1 Rest Period: 45 seconds to 1 minute between exercises				No. of sets: 2
	Double Arm Swing, Step-Step	64	25	15
Swing Snatch, Overhead Squat		63, 91	20	12 each
Drill 2 Rest Period: 45 seconds to 1 minute between exercises				No. of sets: 2
	Romanian Dead Lift	73	25	12
	Single Arm Swing	60	20	12 each
Drill 3 Rest Period: 45 seconds to 1 minute between exercises				No. of sets: 2
	Stay in Squat Figure 8	78	25	12 each

PLATINUM PROGRAM, Week 4, Wednesday				
	Exercise	**Page #**	**Weight**	**No. of Reps**
	Torso Circles	94	25	12 each
Drill 4				
Rest Period: up to 45 seconds between exercises			No. of sets: 2	
	Russian Twist (feet crossed and elevated)	98	20	15
Cool Down/Stretch				

PLATINUM PROGRAM, Week 4, Friday				
	Exercise	**Page #**	**Weight**	**No. of Reps**
Warm-up				
Drill 1				
Rest Period: 30 to 45 seconds after two exercises are completed			No. of sets: 2	
	Overhead Press, Elbow to Knee	79	15	15
	Single Arm Swing	60	20	10 each then switch hands 10 each

PLATINUM PROGRAM, Week 4, Friday				
	Exercise	**Page #**	**Weight**	**No. of Reps**
Drill 2 Rest Period: 30 to 45 seconds after two exercises are completed			No. of sets: 2	
	Lateral Lunge, Open Arm	54	15	10 each
	One Legged Dead Lift with Kettlebell	75	20	10 each
Drill 3 Rest Period: 30 to 45 seconds after two exercises are completed			No. of sets: 2	
	Side Plank Row, Pass	101	20	8 each
	Clam	102	15	15
Cool Down/Stretch				

PLATINUM PROGRAM, Week 4, Saturday				
Warm-up				
Drill 1 Rest Period: up to 90 seconds			No. of sets: 3	
Swing Snatch to Windmill with Overhead Kettlebell		63, 89	20	4 minutes (alternate sides, 1 minute each, no less than 8 reps per minute)

	Exercise	Page #	Weight	No. of Reps
PLATINUM PROGRAM, Week 4, Saturday				
Drill 2				
Rest Period: up to 45 seconds between drills			No. of sets: 3	
	Squat/Stand Figure 8	77	20	1 minute
Cool Down/Stretch				

	Exercise	Page #	Weight	No. of Reps
PLATINUM PROGRAM, Week 5, Monday				
Warm-up				
Drill 1				
Rest Period: up to 1 minute after 2 exercises are completed			No. of sets: 2	
	Halo	51	20	8 each
	Vertical Clean, Press	83, 49	20	15 each
Drill 2				
Rest Period: up to 1 minute after 2 exercises are completed			No. of sets: 2	
	Single Arm Swing with Hand Switch	62	20	15 each

PLATINUM PROGRAM, Week 5, Monday				
	Exercise	**Page #**	**Weight**	**No. of Reps**
	Single Arm High Pull with Switches	69	20	10 each

Drill 3
Rest Period: up to 1 minute after 2 exercises are completed   No. of sets: 2

	Lateral Lunge, Open Arm	54	15	15
	Swing to Right Angle, Bottom Up	80	20	15 each

Drill 4
Rest Period: up to 1 minute after 2 exercises are completed   No. of sets: 2

	Plank Row, Pass	100	20	10
	Overhead/Chest/Situp/Press	99	15	15

Cool Down/Stretch

PLATINUM PROGRAM, Week 5, Wednesday				
	Exercise	**Page #**	**Weight**	**No. of Reps**
Warm-up				
Drill 1				
Rest Period: 45 seconds to 1 minute after 2 exercises are completed			No. of sets: 3	
	Overhead Squat	91	15	10 each
	Double Arm Swing	58	25	12
Drill 2				
Rest Period: up to 90 seconds			No. of sets: 1	
	Full Turkish Get Up	92	15	5 each
Drill 3				
Rest Period: 45 seconds to 1 minute after 2 exercises are completed			No. of sets: 3	
	Romanian Dead Lift	73	25	12
	Forward Walking Lunge	53	15	15

PLATINUM PROGRAM, Week 5, Wednesday				
	Exercise	**Page #**	**Weight**	**No. of Reps**
Drill 4 Rest Period: up to 90 seconds				No. of sets: 1
	Full Turkish Get Up	92	15	5 each
Drill 5 Rest Period: 45 seconds to 1 minute after 2 exercises are completed				No. of sets: 3
	Overhead Press, Elbow to Knee	79	15	10 each
	Stay in Squat Figure 8	78	25	10
Drill 6 Rest Period: 45 seconds to 1 minute after 2 exercises are completed				No. of sets: 2
	Russian Twist (feet crossed and elevated)	98	15	25
Cool Down/Stretch				

PLATINUM PROGRAM, Week 5, Friday				
	Exercise	**Page #**	**Weight**	**No. of Reps**
Warm-up				
Drill 1				
Rest Period: 45 seconds to 1 minute between exercises			No. of sets: 3	
	Single Arm Swing	60	20	10 each then switching hands 10 each
	Swing Clean, Push Press, Two Kettlebell Windmill*	85, 90	20	8, 6, 4
	Swing Snatch	63	20	15 each
	Side Plank Row	101	20	10 each
	Clam	102	20	10
	Russian Twist (feet crossed and elevated)	98	20	15
Cool Down/Stretch				

* Images should be read clock-wise.

PLATINUM PROGRAM, Week 5, Saturday				
	Exercise	**Page #**	**Weight**	**Time**
Warm-up				
Drill 1 Rest Period: 30 seconds			No. of sets: 3	
	Double Arm Swing	58	25	1 minute
Drill 2 Rest Period: up to 2 minutes			No. of sets: 3	
	Swing Clean	82	25	4 minutes (alternate arms every 30 seconds, no less than 10 reps per 30 seconds)
Drill 3 Rest Period: up to 30 seconds			No. of sets: 3	
	Push Up (straight legs)	76	n/a	30 seconds (no less than 10 reps in 30 seconds)
Cool Down/Stretch				

PLATINUM PROGRAM, Week 6, Monday				
	Exercise	**Page #**	**Weight**	**No. of Reps**
Warm-up				
Drill 1 Rest Period: 45 seconds to 1 minute between exercises			No. of sets: 3	
	Double Arm Swing	58	25	15

PLATINUM PROGRAM, Week 6, Monday					
	Exercise		**Page #**	**Weight**	**No. of Reps**
Swing Snatch to Overhead Squat			63, 91	20	10 each
Drill 2 Rest Period: 45 seconds to 1 minute between exercises				No. of sets: 3	
	Romanian Dead Lift		73	25	15
	Single Arm Swing		60	20	15 each
Drill 3 Rest Period: up to 90 seconds between exercises				No. of sets: 2	
	Full Turkish Get Up		92	20	4 each
Drill 4 Rest Period: 45 seconds to 1 minute between exercises				No. of sets: 2	
	Stay in Squat Figure 8		78	20	10 each

Body Sculpting *with* **Kettlebells**

PLATINUM PROGRAM, Week 6, Monday				
	Exercise	**Page #**	**Weight**	**No. of Reps**
	Torso Circles	94	25	10 each
Drill 5				
Rest Period: 45 seconds to 1 minute between exercises			**No. of sets: 2**	
	Russian Twist (feet crossed and elevated)	98	20	20
Cool Down/Stretch				

PLATINUM PROGRAM, Week 6, Wednesday				
	Exercise	**Page #**	**Weight**	**No. of Reps**
Warm-up				
Drill 1				
Rest Period: 30 to 45 seconds between exercises			**No. of sets: 3**	
	Single Arm Swing	60	20	10 each then switching hands 10 each
		82, 49, 90	20	12, 8, 6
Swing Clean, Press, Two Kettlebell Windmill				
	One Legged Dead Lift with Kettlebell	75	20	12, 8, 6

* Images should be read clock-wise.

PLATINUM PROGRAM, Week 6, Wednesday				
	Exercise	**Page #**	**Weight**	**No. of Reps**
	Russian Twist (feet crossed and elevated)	98	15	25
	Clam	102	15	15
Cool Down/Stretch				

PLATINUM PROGRAM, Week 6, Friday				
	Exercise	**Page #**	**Weight**	**No. of Reps**
Warm-up				
Drill 1				
Rest Period: 30 to 45 seconds between exercises				No. of sets: 3
	Hanging Straight Arm Squat to Vertical Clean, Push Press*	47, 85	20	10 each
	Single Arm Swing, Swing Clean (1 Swing + 1 Clean = 1 rep)	60, 82	20	10 each
Drill 2				
Rest Period: 30 to 45 seconds between exercises				No. of sets: 3
	Swing Snatch	63	20	12 each

PLATINUM PROGRAM, Week 6, Friday				
	Exercise	**Page #**	**Weight**	**No. of Reps**
	Side Plank Row, Pass	101	20	10 each
Drill 3 Rest Period: up to 90 seconds between exercises				No. of sets: 2
	Full Turkish Get Up	92	20	5 each
Cool Down/Stretch				

PLATINUM PROGRAM, Week 6, Saturday				
	Exercise	**Page #**	**Weight**	**Time**
Warm-up				
Drill 1				No. of sets: 1
	Swing Snatch (rest up to 5 minutes)	63	20	6 minutes (alternate arms every minute, no less than 14 reps per minute)
	Single Arm High Pull with Switches (rest up to 30 seconds)	69	20	30 seconds
	Russian Twist (feet crossed and elevated; rest up to 1 minute)	98	20	30 seconds

PLATINUM PROGRAM, Week 6, Saturday				
	Exercise	**Page #**	**Weight**	**Time**
Drill 2				No. of sets: 1
	Swing Snatch (rest up to 5 minutes)	63	20	6 minutes (alternate arms every minute, no less than 14 reps per minute)
	Single Arm High Pull with Switches (rest up to 30 seconds)	69	20	30 seconds
	Russian Twist (feet crossed and elevated; rest up to 1 minute)	98	20	30 seconds
Cool Down/Stretch				

Appendix

It is natural to have many questions when it comes to any new idea or training concept being learned, and it is certainly no surprise that many people, when first introduced to kettlebells, are curious.

Here are a few of the most common questions and concerns.

Are kettlebells dangerous?
Unusual perhaps, but kettlebells are actually less dangerous than any other training device or weight when utilized properly. As with any fitness tool or regimen, it's all about following procedures and learning proper technique. When you observe the unique circular movements allowed by the kettlebell, you will notice its similarity to every day activities: swinging your purse over your shoulder, lifting a child, walking a lunging dog or carrying grocery bags.

Kettlebells actually cause less injury than most other fitness modalities and this book will teach you specifically how to move the bell properly. By using guidelines found within this book, safety should not become an issue.

Will it hurt my back?
This is a very common misconception but easily put to rest. Because all the kettlebell movements are initiated from the hips and not the spine, the back is actually a stabilizing factor, not a prime mover. When the kettlebell is in motion, the body will naturally respond, much like a reflex, to stabilize itself. This reflex reaction enables the spinal muscles, both superficial and deep, to engage, supporting your entire body throughout the movements.

The majority of the moves are performed in a standing position, which is the optimal position for full-body engagement and injury prevention.

I haven't worked out in years, so can I begin with kettlebells?
Yes, kettlebells are a great training tool for getting back into shape after a long lay-off or even after pregnancy. You will reap more significant results in less time than you ever imagined!

Will these weights make me bulky and too muscular?
Another unfortunate misconception!

Kettlebell lifting creates bodies that are incredibly strong and lean. Your body's muscle groups will all be engaged at one time, thereby raising your metabolism and burning unwanted fat. The result is a firm, round shape, enhancing your curves while reducing your waistline.

Will these weights be too heavy for me?
The suggested weight for each exercise should not be confused with other resistance tools such as dumbbells or medicine balls. A 15 lb. kettlebell is not the same as a 15 lb. dumbbell and you will notice the difference as soon as you begin moving it, this is when the 'real feel' becomes apparent. Just as we consider the weather in terms of actual temperature and the 'real feel', the actual weight of kettlebells differs from their 'real feel'. The 'real feel' of a 15 lb kettlebell in motion is only 5 or 6 lbs!

This difference in weight will be realized with any object that possesses a displaced center of gravity: take a large purse and create a gentle swinging motion on the outside of your leg. You will immediately notice its lightness due to the presence of momentum.

This is where the kettlebell magic exists—the work is not just in the lifting or moving alone, but also in controlling the movement.

Can't I move the kettlebell like a dumbbell?
You can! Using the kettlebell for two-dimensional movements (such as bicep curls, lateral raises, or simply holding them while performing squats) will indeed be more challenging than using dumbbells because of the kettlebell's displaced center of gravity. But why limit yourself to two-dimensional planes?

This book will be your guide to the skill of kettlebell movements, which are by nature circular, not linear.

Kettlebell Buying Guide
For my selection of the best kettlebells on the market today, please visit my website:

www.lornakleidman.com

Index